Also by Bruce Henderson:

Oakland Organic, Caboose Press, Berkeley 1982 and Albany 1985

A Vegan Primer

Bruce Henderson D.A., M.A.

ILLUSTRATION CREDITS
All drawings by Bruce Henderson except:

For the chapters Personal Experience, Reasons for Vegetarianism, Nutritional Tips: Licia Wolf
For Food Horror Stories: Bob Aul
For Broth: Tamar Brott
For Exercise and Extras, "Jogger" by Jody Keene and "Yoga" by Licia Wolf
For Dairy Products and Spices from Clker.com

ISBN: 978-1-4834-3877-1 (sc)
ISBN: 978-1-4834-3876-4 (e)

Lulu Publishing Services rev. date: 01/15/2016

For my wife Angela and for all those who persist in
trying to build a better human community

Message to Readers

This book does not claim to offer any cure for diseases or ailments, chronic or otherwise. The author cannot be responsible for any ill effects due to dietary change, or to use of foods or other products mentioned in the text. Readers requiring extensive health treatment should seek the guidance of a doctor or naturopath versed in nutritional therapy.

Contents

Preface

This book was originally published in the 1980s under the title *Oakland Organic*. At that time I lived in Oakland, across the bay from San Francisco, and had been changing my diet toward vegetarianism over a number of years. I was also supporting a surge in interest in organic foods, a topic that will be discussed in detail in this book. 100 years ago 40% of Americans were farmers, and most of our food was organic by default since we had yet to develop the artificial fertilizers, petrochemical insecticides and chemical food additives that we have since served ourselves in a kind of chemical feast. Today, according to the American Farm Bureau Federation, just 2% of Americans are farmers. Much of what stocks the supermarket shelves now is the result of "agribusiness," or farming by large corporations such as Cargill, Monsanto, ConAgra and Archer Daniels Midland.

The problem for those interested in better diet 40 years ago, and continuing now, is how, particularly for people who do not have land to grow food themselves, to maximize the nutritional content and health benefits of what we eat. Ideally all Americans would have access to fresh, locally-grown, affordable organic foods. In some ways that goal has become easier than it was 40 years ago, when people had to seek out little independent health food stores and co-ops to buy better foods. Today an increasing number of farmers markets serve urban dwellers and, lest they lose customers to Whole Foods or other health store outlets, even supermarkets now routinely stock organic foods and other items such as soy milk and meat substitutes.

Many Americans settle for convenience over health when it comes to food choices. We have, since the 1950s, succumbed to the culture of "fast food," in a misguided effort to "save time." Many workers get a half-hour lunch during which they rush to a drive-through window, order greasy, high-calorie food, and then eat behind the wheel on their way back to the workplace. Our supermarkets are full of canned, frozen, sometimes irradiated, artificially preserved or otherwise "embalmed" foods. Studies such as Eric Schlosser's *Fast Food Nation* detail the frightening outcomes of our massive system which involves raising animals on feedlots and administering doses of growth hormones and antibiotics; unsafe practices at slaughterhouses; e coli contamination of meat which leads to recalls, food poisoning and sometimes death; and additional health risks introduced by minimum-wage fast food workers in the kitchen and behind the counter of the fast food outlets.

The United States is experiencing an epidemic of obesity. Today, the Centers for Disease Control and Prevention reports 35% of American adults as obese, and 17% of American children. The Organization for Economic Co-operation and Development estimates that 3/4 of the American population will likely be overweight or obese by 2020. Particularly since the advent and proliferation of fast food outlets the American obesity rate has steadily climbed. There is also speculation that the growth hormones and antibiotics which are given to animals to boost their weight gain are also contributing to weight gain in the people who consume those animals.

Beyond concerns about being overweight, an ongoing study funded by the National Institutes of Health demonstrates that vegetarians live on average almost eight years longer than the general population, similar to the gap between smokers and nonsmokers. An involuntary experiment in vegetarianism for an entire population happened during World Wars I and II, when wartime food restrictions mostly eliminated meat consumption in Scandinavian countries. A significant decline in the mortality rate followed, which only returned to prewar levels after the restriction was lifted.

There are also everyday benefits including a feeling of better health on the part of vegetarians. A study of 15,000 American vegetarians determined that those who eat meat have twice the odds of being on antacids, aspirin, blood pressure medications, insulin, laxatives, painkillers, sleeping pills, and tranquilizers. So plant-based diets can help people avoid taking drugs, paying for drugs, or risking adverse side effects (*Huffington Post*, 12/26/12).

Chapters to follow will further explain why you might wish to avoid meat in your diet, and explain ways to gradually transition to healthier fare.

Vegetarianism as a philosophy and practice dates back thousands of years. Over the centuries, those seeking higher spiritual consciousness also embraced vegetarianism in the belief that a healthier body leads to a healthier state of mind. There is also the idea of optimal health; that health is not simply the absence of disease or pain, but the enjoyment of the higher functioning of both body and mind.

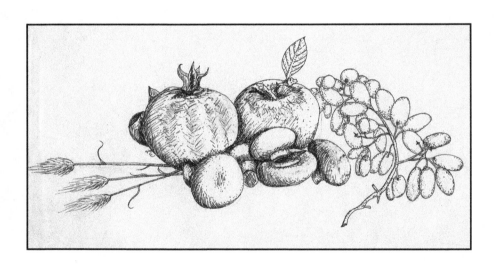

Personal Experience

The first realization that pointed me in the direction of vegetarianism was basic: that what we eat affects our health. That may seem intuitive, yet judging by the amount of "junk foods" and fast foods Americans consume, there are many who have not grasped this fundamental principle. The proverbial "you are what you eat" is worth considering. Most of the cells in your body renew and replace themselves every 7 to 10 years; the surface layer of skin (epidermis) recycles every two weeks! Red blood cells change out every two months, and liver cells every year. So if your body is constantly regenerating and growing new cells, you want to ask yourself how well you are nourishing your body so that it can do this vital work well—so that your body has the best materials to work with.

In the now-classic film *Supersize Me*, Morgan Spurlock experiments on himself by eating only meals from McDonalds for one month. Starting out in good health and monitored by three physicians, Spurlock gains weight, loses energy, often feels sick, and well before the month is out, gets warned by one of his doctors that if he doesn't end his experiment he may suffer permanent liver damage. The clear indication is that not only was fast food not nourishing his body very well, it was actually damaging his health. Certainly one person does not represent a scientific sample, and most people don't go to McDonalds for all of their meals. But if you are eating daily or frequent fast food meals on a regular basis, you have to ask yourself what that may be doing to your body over a span of years, and whether your health wouldn't be better if you gave your body healthier fare to work with.

There are a variety of reasons why people may adopt vegetarianism, including sympathy for the animals slaughtered to provide meat; concern for the environment due to stress on resources and other damages which

1

result from a meat-based culture; existing health problems associated with high-fat, high-cholesterol or high-protein intake from animal foods; or even spiritual or religious beliefs. None of these was my primary motivation. I became vegetarian out of fear of the eventual consequences if I did not. Once I understood that the foods I chose determined the outcomes for my health, I started reading and researching in earnest, which I have continued to do ever since. The more I learned about meat processing, the dairy industry, agribusiness, and alternatives, the more concerned I became and the more motivated to find a healthier way to go.

One other key concept to becoming vegetarian is that as you give up animal products, you will want to find the most nutritious versions of plant foods that you can. For example, if you are going to eat rice, you will want to avoid processed white rice and instead prepare brown rice which has many nutritional advantages. Here we get into the issue of fast food again; yes, it usually takes more time to cook brown rice that it does to use white minute-rice. (Though even that is changing. Trader Joe's stores sell precooked brown rice packets that can be microwaved and ready in 3 minutes if you really are in a hurry). But isn't your health worth the extra time it may take to prepare food? Why "save" a few minutes a day by settling for processed quick foods when you may actually be taking years off your life? And what are you saving the time for? Is anything worth more than your health?

A goal should be to obtain organic, fresh produce whenever possible. Farmers markets sell locally-grown fruits and vegetables, and rising demand for organic foods has resulted in more and more stores and supermarkets stocking them on their shelves. The idea is to choose plant foods that offer the most nutrition with the fewest residues of pesticides, chemicals, artificial colors, genetically modified organisms and the like.

While you might want to make a clean break from animal foods, a step-by-step transition will likely prove easier because it will give you time to adjust and time to learn how to substitute nutritionally for the foods you are giving up. When I was growing up I had a pretty typical American diet for the times. Fast food had not yet become a common practice for families. Items we are used to now such as whole wheat bread or soy foods were hard to come by. But my mother did a lot of "scratch" cooking of decent foods. She made sure her family got a balanced intake which included fresh fruits, vegetables, grains and proteins. She would send us around the corner to buy produce from a local farm stand. But the family meals also included canned and processed food, meat and fish, milk and eggs. I suffered from the typical ailments that went along with such a diet, whether from food prepared at home or from similar choices elsewhere: constipation, upset stomach, acne, and occasional mild food poisoning. I also experienced bouts of serious ear infections that may well have been diet-related.

I was in my mid-twenties when I decided to give up red meat as a start. There are widely available meat substitutes to transition away from beef, pork, bacon and the like. Probably the biggest hurdle beyond changing one's personal habits is the reaction from friends and family. Even now you will find that many people believe you need to eat meat to be healthy and strong. Your own mother may try to undermine your resolve. But you can find lots of books, articles and websites to encourage you and to reassure you in your decision.

The next step was giving up chicken and fish. Those are animals, not vegetables. While eating poultry may be better nutritionally than eating beef and pork, unfortunately chickens and turkeys are subjected to the same commercial feedlot operations that ultimately make meat a poor choice. (Examples will come in the chapter entitled "Food Horror Stories"). Fish can be a better nutritional choice than either meat or poultry, but there are problems with mercury contamination and with the growing practice of commercial fish farming. If you look in the seafood case of most supermarkets you will see some selections labeled as "Wild Caught." While those may be better choices than the farmed fish, they will be expensive, mercury remains an issue, and in general people are depleting wild fisheries worldwide so making wild-caught fish a frequent choice for meals further stresses the natural environment. Mainstream consumer agencies and the National Resources Defense Council advise parents to avoid giving their kids tuna more than once per week.

Here we reach the dividing line between vegetarianism and veganism. I felt so much better after giving up meat, chicken and fish that one fine spring day I decided to stop using dairy products as well. There are medical and nutritional reasons supporting such a change which this book will review in the chapter on "Dairy Products." First I stopped drinking milk, then stopped eating cheese, and then finally gave up dairy yogurt as well. I even gave up ice cream! (Many vegan substitutes for dairy foods are now readily available such as soy yogurt, almond and rice cheeses, frozen desserts made of almond, soy or rice milk and so forth). With this transition came a two-week period with symptoms resembling a cold with copious drainage: I spit up thick mucus for a fortnight, lost about 5 pounds and felt as if a weight had been lifted from me. The human body is resilient and given half a chance will take the opportunity to rid itself of harmful, congesting residues, recover from smoking and other addictions, and rebuild its strength.

Once I found out how commercial egg-laying hens are treated I also gave up eggs. Such treatment, detailed in the "Food Horror Stories" chapter, made me feel sorry for the hens and fearful for my own health should I continue to eat eggs, particularly from battery hen-houses. Occasionally I will use eggs for cooking, but fortunately consumers can find cage-free, naturally-fed choices in stores. Even those eggs are far from ideal when it comes to questions of animal cruelty, however. "Hard-core" vegans strongly motivated by considerations of how animals are treated will go so far as to try to avoid leather clothing and other consumer goods containing animal products, though to live 100% animal-free represents a difficult challenge for most people. After publishing the first edition of *Oakland Organic* I received a letter from a reader chastising me for recommending bee pollen as a food since, according to the correspondent, bees can sometimes lose one of their legs when going through the tiny brushes which remove the pollen as they return to their hives. So in this case concern for animal welfare extended even to insects!

Overall I felt much better leaving animal products behind. Setting matters of conscience aside, physically I experienced renewed surges of energy to the point where I took up marathon running. Before becoming vegetarian I often felt sluggish, sometimes constipated, regularly experienced heartburn and sour stomach and many minor-league ailments that seemed to vanish as I left my former eating habits behind. Staying at a healthy weight became much easier, and I even felt more clear-headed. I also found little need for aspirin, stomach antacids, laxatives and other over-the-counter remedies for ailments which can be linked to diet in the first place.

I have now followed a vegetarian diet for decades and it has clearly served me well. Certainly individuals are different in their size and shape, predisposition for certain illnesses, metabolism and other considerations related to physical make-up. But at a stage of life when I have reached average retirement age, I still enjoy the energy to raise two children and to play soccer several times a week, very different outcomes from what would have been thought of as normal a generation ago. By my age my own father suffered from arthritis, high blood pressure and prostate cancer and could no longer even go bowling. Yet I have kept a clean bill of health on all of those fronts. I have maintained a consistent weight for decades, so that I can keep clothes until they wear out rather than expecting to buy increasingly larger sizes as time goes on. Best of all, on a day to day basis I have enjoyed good health and have avoided much suffering from ailments and "dis-ease" that follow poor food choices.

We have also elected to raise our twin girls as vegetarians. Certainly when they reach age 18 and wish to choose for themselves they can adopt any diet they want. But so far they are proud to be vegetarians and have enjoyed good health and normal growth. They are both active with soccer and gymnastics as well as their schoolwork in addition to a full social life. When friends offer meat they refuse; for that matter when we are with company who are eating meat and we, their parents, ask if they want to try it, they decline. We have pet rabbits, and the twins love animals (as most children do), but they are not caught in the dilemma of "loving animals" and then eating them anyway. They could not imagine eating the rabbits, which they treat as friends. They enjoy soymilk, veggie burgers, "fake" bacon and "fake" sausage made of soy and other similar foods because that's what they are used to and have been raised eating and what they see their parents eating. Interestingly many of their friends, when eating with us, enjoy these same foods and also take them in stride, never complaining that they don't taste good or that they want something else.

Tips:

For people raised on a "normal" diet, changing long-held patterns of eating may take considerable time. It may be most effective to spread the changes out over a long period so that gains are assimilated gradually. Trying to make a radical change all at once may result in backsliding or giving up because it seems too difficult or too different from what you were used to. Many accounts of dietary change talk about a "cleansing reaction," so that you may feel a bit worse before you feel better and healthier. That could be due to toxins, now being more efficiently expelled since you are no longer introducing new doses of them into your body, entering your bloodstream and temporarily dragging down your feelings of well-being.

You may find that FASTING for a day or two or even longer can help with such detoxifying of your system. A separate chapter on fasting is included in this book. When I got serious about changing my diet I successfully undertook a fast of 20 days with no apparent harm. Remember too that health is holistic. That means that paying attention to diet is only a part of seeking better health. Exercise, in whatever form you choose, is almost universally recommended by every type of health care practitioner. (There are more details in the chapter "Exercise and Extras"). You may also find that practicing yoga and meditation help you to not only keep your body limber, but to connect you, even in a modest way, to the spiritual side of the improvements you are trying to make. Resting, napping and trying to avoid stress will also aid you in making a significant changeover.

If what you are trying to do seems unusual, unfamiliar or radical, it is worth noting that people will locate themselves along a scale of dietary practices. On one end are those who give no thought to what they eat, and do not concern themselves with the quality of their food. Somewhere in the middle are people like my own mom who stick to mainstream food choices while trying to maintain a well-balanced variety of foods. Then there are those who adopt the various diets we hear about: Paleo, Atkins, Weight Watchers, South Beach, Pritikin and others on a long list. Beyond those groups come the vegetarians who give up beef and pork, poultry and fish but may still use some animal products. Then come the vegans who avoid all animal products. But there are also those who seek to eat only raw foods, and even fruitarians! Given all these variations, some of which seem off in some extreme corner, you need not feel too self-conscious about making some changes. A 2013 Public Policy Polling survey found 13% of Americans identify as vegetarian, so such a choice is no longer considered unusual.

Here are some tips to save you time and trouble on your way:

1. Get rid of or give away foods that reinforce bad habits. Purge your cupboards of junky snack foods containing loads of salt, sugar and preservatives; sugary breakfast cereals; donuts, cookies and similar packaged prepared desserts except as use for occasional treats; candy and other foods that represent "empty calories;" most frozen or canned vegetables if fresh versions are readily

available; foods mostly made with beached white flour including frozen pizzas, breads and pastries; old boxes of packaged cake and pancake mixes.

2. Other items to reconsider:

- Salt, at least if you have been in the habit of liberally tossing it over everything on your plate. With better food choices you will learn to appreciate the actual food flavors themselves
- Very salty condiments such as steak sauce (especially since you won't be eating any more steak!)
- Crisco and other hydrogenated and solid shortenings, and of course lard; vegetable oils will be much better choices
- Preserved meat products including jerky, cold cuts, frankfurters, liverwurst; which the food writer John Callela referred to as "imitation flesh foods put together from the waste and septic parts of the animal"
- Sugary sodas and soft drinks; recently a 16-year-old high school girl discovered that Gatorade contained flame retardant as an ingredient to maintain uniform color. After a successful online petition parent company Pepsico removed this brominated vegetable oil from Gatorade, but not from its Mountain Dew product since no one specifically complained about that drink
- Foods that contain or call for loads of sugar: Kool-Aid, fruit juices that are mostly water and sugar; fruits canned in heavy syrups, corn syrups and overly-sugary jams and jellies (fruit is naturally sweet, and you can find unsweetened or lightly sweetened versions of jams, applesauce and apple butter, etc.)

Restock your kitchen and pantry with fresh, whole foods. The idea here is that if you want a snack and your choice is either fresh grapes that you have on hand, or trekking to the store to buy cookies, you will likely snack on the fresh fruit, and will have plenty of time to reconsider any lingering impulses to "junk out" on preserved "frankenfoods." In this way purging your kitchen will help you get past old addictions and learn to appreciate healthier, more natural foods.

Again following advice from the writer John Callela, here are foods most desirable in the diet:

1st- class food: fresh fruits, nuts, vegetables, seeds, legumes and tubers grown in nature's garden containing the seven basic nutrients (vitamins, minerals, proteins, carbohydrates, essential fatty acids, enzymes and trace elements). Ideally some of these would be gathered from the wild, benefitting from the sun's energy; next best are the products of organic gardening and farming; then there are hydroponics and indoor sprouted foods.

2nd-class food: Fractured foods prepared and combined without artificial additives or flavors or excessive cooking: unleavened bread, cold-pressed oils, nut and seed butters, vegetable juices and purees.

3rd-class food: fruits and vegetables, nuts, legumes, tubers and grains slightly cooked to enhance their flavors and release some of their nutrients; whole grain breads, steamed or lightly sautéed broccoli, cauliflower or squashes, and fruit preserves. Note that Americans are encouraged to buy frozen vegetables that have already been cooked once before being frozen and packaged, and then are cooked AGAIN before being served. No wonder kids turn up their noses, or else they come drowned in sauces and condiments so that they taste like something. And all that processing kills off many of the nutrients and enzymes that the fresh foods contained in the first place.

For many people giving up meat won't prove too difficult, since meat substitutes such as veggie burgers and veggie hot dogs (and many others) are readily available in stores, supermarkets and restaurants.

Chicken and fish many prove trickier since chicken is a regular staple of sandwiches, salads, wraps and burritos. Many do not really consider chicken and fish to be meat, but they are animal foods and in the case of fish we have unfortunately polluted the waters they swim in with mercury, agricultural runoff, and plastic residues that are now found in most seafood. More discussion of the down side of consuming such foods will follow in later chapters.

As you change your diet toward eating whole foods that yield more nutrition than what you were used to ---say, eating whole wheat bread instead of bread made with puffed-up bleached white flour, or granola instead of Cheerios—you may find yourself eating less. You may find yourself craving fewer snacks between meals since the whole foods should prove to be more satisfying. Remember too that eating is partly about hunger and partly psychological. We eat to celebrate occasions, we eat to reward or to comfort ourselves, we eat out of boredom or anxiety. If you have decided to eat to gain better nutrition, and you "keep your eyes on the prize," you will be less likely to turn to empty snacking either for psychological reasons or because you no longer feel empty or hungry soon after eating foods that don't truly nourish you.

Giving up or cutting back on sweets is also a good idea. We live in a time when one out of three Americans can expect to contract diabetes. In the last 20 years type 2 diabetes, which used to be mostly an adult disease, has become an epidemic among children. Being overweight and not getting enough exercise are typical precursors to type 2 diabetes. Candy, cookies, sugary cereals and other overly-sweetened foods contribute to becoming overweight and undermine the body's nutrition since they are mostly "empty calories." And of course since diabetes is fundamentally the inability of the body to keep blood sugar in balance by producing enough insulin, eating lots of sweets will only tax the body's systems. It's important to remember that donuts may be vegetarian food, but they are hardly the best choice when it comes to health.

Giving up dairy products can be difficult because they are ingredients in many foods and because they are heavily promoted by the dairy industry itself. What is advertised and promoted can come to seem "normal," but that doesn't mean such foods represent the best choices. A separate chapter this book will take up the hazards of dairy consumption in detail, but for now you can measure your own potential resistance to this idea by how frequently you indulge in ice cream, cottage cheese, yogurt, sliced cheese and all the many variations of dairy foods.

In the end each of us is different and you may decide that going meatless works for you but going "vegan" will not. However, once you start down the path of better diet, and start experiencing freedom from previous suffering and disease and increased feelings of well-being, you may gain new incentive to persist in transforming your health by giving up damaging old habits and embracing new and healthier eating. You may discover the difference between feeling "OK" and experiencing optimal health.

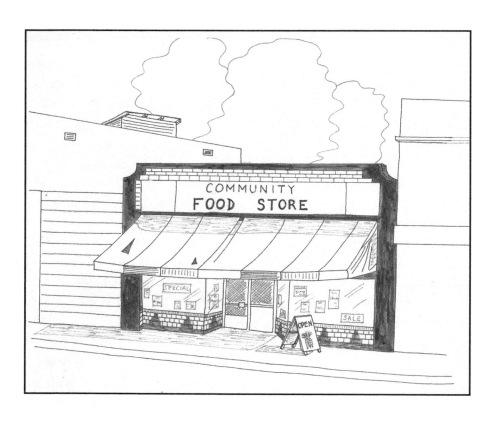

Organic Foods and Holistic Nutrition

The poet Gary Snyder, whose work strongly reflects a concern with nature and our environment, once wrote about riding past an agricultural field and reflecting that, after all, wasn't he really looking out the window at himself? That is, insofar as he might eat what was growing in the field, which would later become part of his own body, wasn't he therefore directly connected to those plants? And so, on reflection, shouldn't we all be concerned about how our food is grown? This would be especially true for vegetarians who eat plants directly, but the truth is that, with the exception of a few odd organisms living on the deep sea floor, most life on our planet depends on photosynthesis. Simply put, a cow is a vegetarian! So even if you eat meat, you ought to be concerned with what the cow is eating. That is why today you will find in the meat case of your local supermarket consumer choices which include "range-fed" beef, meaning animals fed in a more natural way than the more typical practice of the feedlot.

Wine lovers take great concern over the specific region that produced certain grapes that went into a particular batch of wine. The Wikipedia definition of an "appellation" is "a legally defined and protected geographical indication used to identify where the grapes for a wine were grown; other types of food often have appellations as well." Oenophiles clearly believe that the specific climate and soil in which grapes are grown makes a difference. Similarly, there are foods famous for being grown in certain regions, such as Idaho potatoes, cranberries from Massachusetts, chilies from New Mexico, Michigan cherries, Oregon hazelnuts, or California olallieberries. While these crops can be grown in other places, specific regions are recognized as growing the finest produce.

This principle of growing conditions affecting the quality of crops is key to understanding the movement for organic foods. For the vast majority of its history, agriculture was organic more or less by default, since it was only during the 20th century that a large supply of newly-developed chemicals were introduced to the food supply. The organic farming movement arose in the 1940s in response to the industrialization of agriculture known as the Green Revolution. While the intention to feed more people may have been worthy, we have all paid a price for taking this direction with our agriculture. Some of the damage is documented here in the "Food Horror Stories" chapter. When Lincoln was President, 90% of Americans were farmers. By 1900 farmers represented about 40% of the American labor force, with small farms still predominating. Today, just 2% of Americans are farmers, and much of what is grown is now produced by giant corporate agricultural combines, sometimes referred to as "agribusiness."

Our current system practices monocropping, growing vast acreages of a single crop using artificial fertilizers, pesticides sprayed from planes and huge machines. The produce in stores might be from such operations, or could be flown in from other countries where there are even fewer safeguards and regulations over how crops are grown. Contrast that system to a store I once visited in Santa Cruz, California where the bins were labeled with the name and address of farmer who grew that food! That may seem extreme, yet consumers could be assured that the food was locally and responsibly produced, and if dissatisfied, could visit the farmer who grew the food with any complaints.

Organic refers to food that is non-chemically treated, grown without use of unapproved pesticides, and fresh or minimally processed. Organic fruit, for example, would be produced this way and ideally be tree-ripened and grown by a local farmer so that the ripe fruit would not suffer from shipping over long distances. Anyone who has eaten tree-ripened fruit from a backyard vine, bush or tree can appreciate the difference in flavor from supermarket versions of the same fruit. Commercially grown tomatoes are picked while they are still green and hard to make them easier to ship, and then artificially ripened using ethylene gas.

Foods claiming to be organic must be free of artificial food additives, and are often processed with fewer artificial methods, materials and conditions, so as to avoid chemical ripening, food irradiation, and genetically modified ingredients. Pesticides are allowed as long as they are not synthetic. While it has proven hard to verify scientifically that pesticide residues or genetically modified organisms cause harm to humans, such practices certainly cause harm to animals in the ecosystem.

"Intensive monoculture depletes soil and leaves it vulnerable to erosion. Chemical fertilizer runoff and CAFO [concentrated animal feeding operation] wastes add to global warming emissions and create oxygen-deprived "dead zones" at the mouths of major waterways. Herbicides and insecticides harm wildlife and can pose human health risks as well. Biodiversity in and near monoculture fields takes a hit, as populations of birds and beneficial insects decline." *(Union of Concerned Scientists; http://www.ucsusa.org/our-work/ food-agriculture/our-failing-food-system/industrial-agriculture).*

And there is, of course, concern over effects on human health of many of our current farming practices. The American Academy of Environmental Medicine (AAEM) urges doctors to prescribe non-GMO [genetically modified organisms] diets for all patients. They cite animal studies showing organ damage, gastrointestinal and immune system disorders, accelerated aging, and infertility. Human studies show how genetically modified (GM) food can leave material behind inside us, possibly causing long-term problems. Genes inserted into GM soy, for example, can transfer into the DNA of bacteria living inside us. The toxic insecticide produced by GM corn was found in the blood of pregnant women and their unborn fetuses.

The good news is that organic foods are no longer hard to find; three-fourths of supermarkets now carry them. Learning about organic foods and vegetarianism leads to understanding our food system today and to thinking about healthful directions overall, not just for our bodies but for the animals and the world around us. One other useful perspective for those resolving to improve their health through better eating is that better health is a holistic enterprise; diet is only one component. Later chapters in this book will explore the benefits of exercise, yoga, avoiding stress and other integral parts of taking the direction toward optimal health.

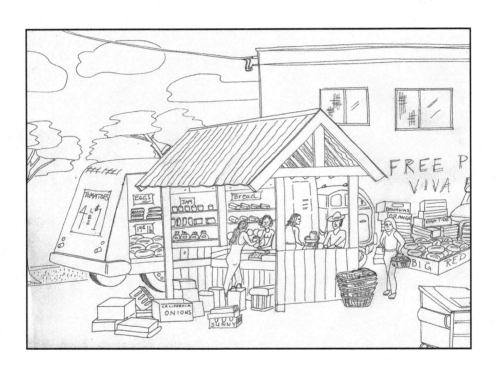

Reasons for Vegetarianism

Humans are omnivores; we are designed to eat almost anything. The Frenchman Michel Lotito ate several bicycles and even a Cessna 150 airplane. Native Americans of the Great Plains ate buffalo, so in whatever other ways we may wish to honor them, they were not vegetarians. (Of course it is worth reflecting that those buffalo traditionally were "grass-fed" and "free-range" animals since we had yet to develop mechanized agriculture). In our time, people living in developed countries can obtain almost any food they desire from around the world. So why should we choose vegetarianism now?

Once answer lies in the horrors of food processing, starting with what is actually done to animals to fulfill the huge demand for meat that is partly driven by promotion by the American Meat Institute and advertising by the fast food industry. The motto of the American Beef Council is "Meat—It's What's for Dinner," and many Americans have come to believe that their meals are not complete, or even lack proper nourishment, without meat. Indeed, the meat lobby has even influenced federal food guidelines such as the "food pyramid" created to guide consumers. In 1977 Senator George McGovern's committee on nutrition created goals that advised Americans to "decrease consumption of meat." But under pressure from meat producers, federal dietary advice evolved into the recommendation, "have two or three daily servings." The meat lobby even demanded and got the color of the saturated fat/cholesterol guideline changed from red to purple because meat producers worried that using red to signify "bad" fat would be linked to red meat in consumers' minds.

We could reason that Americans simply like meat, and that it's a tradition deriving from the natural abundance of the vast continent Europeans began colonizing in 1492. But people are not born with a preference for any particular

15

foods. Food preferences are largely cultural. In Cambodia, fried spiders are a regional delicacy. People in Africa and Indonesia routinely eat termites for protein. Grubs, or beetle larvae, are a high-protein staple of Aboriginal diets in Australia. The native people of Alaska enjoy a concoction made from reindeer fat or tallow, seal oil, freshly fallen snow, and fresh berries called *akutaq* or Eskimo "ice cream." You get the idea. Foods that might disgust average Americans are prized dishes in other cultures.

Similarly, people from other cultures might well be disgusted by a typical American meal of a hamburger and fries. Traditionally the Asian diet has consisted largely of rice and vegetables with a seasoning of meat in small amounts, yet in parts of China life expectancy is greater than in the U. S., and Asian Americans across the board live the longest of any American ethnicity. The American habit of bacon and eggs for breakfast, a hamburger for lunch and steak for dinner has brought along with it heart disease as the number one cause of death in the U. S. and an obesity rate of 35% of adults.

Obviously some people turn to vegetarianism out of concern for animal welfare. Organizations such as People for the Ethical Treatment of Animals provide lots of information on that issue. It can be gut-wrenching to watch a video clip of a sick animal being prodded or pushed by a small bulldozer up the slaughterhouse ramp. That also means that rather than forgo the profits from processing a sick animal, such tainted meat goes into our food supply. It's not easy to separate one concern from another. I have often wondered how kids who participate in 4H clubs and raise farm animals as if they were pets then turn around and sell those same animals for meat at auction. Most kids love animals, which populate the stories they enjoy and take endearing form in the stuffed animals that they hug. And of course most children enjoy having pets and would likely be horrified if anyone proposed serving their pets for dinner.

It is interesting, therefore, to reflect on the fact that we use euphemisms for the meat we consume. We call meat from cows *beef* or *steak*. We call pig meat *pork*. *Veal* refers to the meat of baby cows (calves) slaughtered from just a few days to about 20 weeks old. *Hot dogs* largely consist of meat mush (from rather unappetizing parts of cows, pigs and chickens) mixed with fat, but certainly we hope they do not contain any parts of dogs. And *hamburgers* are made from beef, not ham. *Ham* itself, along with *bacon*, are euphemisms for parts of pigs. There are no animals called a bacon or a ham or a pork. While we actually call turkey meat turkey, and chicken meat chicken, poultry seems to be considered as non-meat somehow, so that the American Heart Association recommends eating more "chicken and fish" than red meat to help avoid heart disease.

Meat in the supermarket comes in neat, shrink-wrapped packages that further distance the consumption of meat products from the slaughtered animals. Here we find parts of various animals sold as wings, breasts, brisket, sirloin, chuck, ribs and so forth. It is a fair bet that many children, and quite a few adults, might not be able to identify which specific animals various cuts of meat come from. On top of all this the fast food industry invents servings of meat such as chicken nuggets, consisting at best of about 50% chicken meat, and the rest fat, blood vessels, nerves, connective tissue and ground bone—animal parts that otherwise would wind up in dog food. Similarly, one of my friends liked frozen breaded fish sticks, but disliked eating any whole fish, as if breading and frying little strips of fish somehow disguised it to make it more palatable and appealing.

There are some who turn to vegetarianism out of concern for our environment. Here is a bracing quote from an article by Malcolm Moore that appeared in the *UK Telegraph* of Oct. 12, 2012: "Leading water scientists have also issued warnings recently that the world may have to switch almost completely to a vegetarian diet over the next 40 years to avoid catastrophic shortages." That is because meat production is water-intensive, requiring much more water than fruits, vegetables or grains. One pound of beef requires 2,000 gallons of water to produce. In contrast, a pound of wheat takes only 138 gallons of water to produce, a pound of corn takes 108 gallons of water, and a pound of soybeans 206 gallons. When it comes to water conservation, why use ten or twenty times the amount of water by feeding corn and soybeans to animals when we could just eat the corn and soybeans directly, thereby not only saving precious water, but feeding more people in the process? When you do the math, pound for pound we could feed 10 to 15 people bread and tofu using the same resources taken to feed beef to just one person. If a 1,000-pound cow yields 600 pounds of beef, that cow used 1.5 million gallons of water and 7,800 pounds of grain. Or put another way, you could effectively feed thousands of people with the grain and water it takes to produce one cow.

Most animals raised today for slaughter live on factory farms, legally labelled as concentrated animal feeding operations (CAFOs for short). A 2006 report by the Food and Agriculture Organization for the UN estimated that around 18 percent of worldwide human-caused greenhouse gasses aggravating global warming emissions were the result of livestock. A 2009 study for World Watch Institute estimated that figure was actually closer to 50 percent, once undercounted emissions from respiration, land use, and methane were taken into consideration. The Environmental Protection Agency estimates that runoff (which it regulates) from factory farms into waterways is the largest single pollutant in the U. S. Livestock also drink about half of the country's potable water each year, and they produce more excrement than humans, waste which is usually just spread on the ground, further contaminating the water. Their waste also contains antibiotic residue from feedlot operations, which will be detailed later in this book.

"On most factory farms, animals are crowded into relatively small areas; their manure and urine are funneled into massive waste lagoons. These cesspools often break, leak or overflow, sending dangerous microbes, nitrate pollution and drug-resistant bacteria into water supplies. Factory-farm lagoons also emit toxic gases such as ammonia, hydrogen sulfide and methane. What's more, the farms often spray the manure onto land, ostensibly as fertilizer -- these "sprayfields" bring still more of these harmful substances into our air and water." (*Natural Resources Defense Council; http://www.nrdc.org/ water/pollution/nspills.asp*). People who live near or work at factory farms breathe in hundreds of gases which are formed as manure decomposes. The stench can be unbearable, but worse still the gases contain many harmful chemicals. Animal waste also contaminates drinking water supplies. Nitrates often seep from lagoons and sprayfields into groundwater. Drinking water contaminated with nitrates can increase the risk of blue baby syndrome and cause deaths in infants. High levels of nitrates in drinking water near hog factories have also been linked to spontaneous abortions. Several disease outbreaks related to drinking water have been traced to bacteria and viruses from waste. In short, most of us probably wouldn't want to live near, or especially downwind, for a commercial hog farm!

One other environmental consideration concerns the shipping of foods. Americans have come to expect a cornucopia of foods from around the world year-round in their supermarkets. In the era of small farms people used to eat foods in season and lacked the means to ship foods long-distance. The advent of railroads, refrigeration, long-distance trucking and chemical food processing and preservation brought us the "convenience" of a great variety of foods shipped to stores near us, but reflect for a moment on the amount of fuel and the resultant pollution caused by shipping foods worldwide via ships, planes, trains and trucks. While we want to enjoy the benefits of "progress," much of the damage to the environment could be alleviated by seeking out fresher foods from local growers via farmers markets and local offerings in stores, and even growing some food yourself, and certainly too from avoiding the purchase of fast food which is the epitome of processed and shipped food.

Lastly, it is worth mentioning spiritual concerns here. The folk phrase is "you are what you eat," but the idea that food has influence on our thoughts and outlook is not new. If you visited a monastery, wouldn't you be shocked to discover the monks ordering pepperoni pizza and meatball sandwiches delivered for their evening meal? We assume that part of their quest for spiritual growth involves discipline when it comes to food, and eating simply. I remember reading a fable concerning a spiritual master whose refined and simplified diet consisted largely of brown rice, bread and tea. During a festival at their monastery when many guests were invited, they served a banquet of rich foods including chicken, cream, sweets and so forth. Yet the master joined in at the feast, shocking the novices by openly eating the rich foods. Afterward, they queried him as to why he did not stick to his usual simple and austere diet. His reply: "Just for this one evening, I thought I'd get down on your level." "Eat light, feel light" is another instructive phrase. Many believe that eating purer, more simply prepared and more nutritious foods leads to clearer thought and even expanded consciousness.

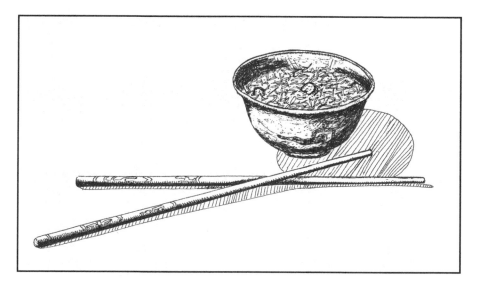

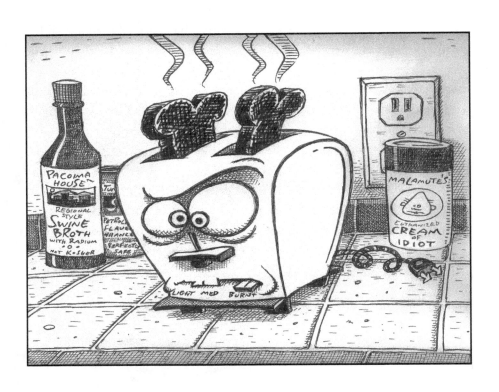

Food Horror Stories

Under the best circumstances, food is prepared to please and nourish those who consume it. If you are preparing food for your family, you probably use the best ingredients you can afford and prepare the food carefully and with love. Certainly you would avoid knowingly poisoning your friends and loved ones. But the outlook changes when providing food turns into agribusiness run by transnational conglomerates. About 10 corporations own most of the food products we buy such as Nestle, Proctor & Gamble, Johnson & Johnson, Unilever and Monsanto. It isn't difficult to find examples of how these large companies often put profit before people. Nestle, for one, has been the target of repeated international boycotts for promoting infant formula over natural breastfeeding in developing countries which has resulted in health issues and death among infants. Some "alternative" and organic foods are likewise owned by familiar parent companies; Coke owns Odwalla, Pepsi owns Naked, and Kraft owns Boca Burgers. As the Consumerist website remarks, "Just because it's organic doesn't mean it was made on a happy communal love-farm."

There is a long history of scandals surrounding food processing in the U.S., going back to at least 100 years ago when Upton Sinclair documented outrageous abuses in the meat-packing industry in his book *The Jungle*. Sinclair's findings led to the passage of the first Pure Food and Drug Act and the Meat Inspection Act of 1906, eventually leading to the establishment of the Food and Drug Administration to oversee the food industry. Unfortunately, as subsequent examples will demonstrate, today's public cannot rely on federal agencies to protect them. An instructive study is Jim Turner's 1970 book *The Chemical Feast*, a Ralph Nader Study Group report. Turner details the "revolving door" of personnel between government agencies and the very industries they are supposed to be regulating. During the 1990s the Clinton Administration found that the meat industry still had the same inspection system it had at the time of the publication of *The Jungle*. As reported by PBS, when Michael Taylor, a lawyer by training who didn't have a meat-industry background, became the new head of the Food Safety and Inspection Service (FSIS), the United States Department of Agriculture's meat-inspection arm, he was surprised at what he found in his new office. "On the telephone there were two speed dials with names by them. And one was to the American Meat Institute and the other was to the National Cattlemen's Association." The meat industry resists effective regulation by contributing heavily to politicians who block reform legislation, by lobbying, and by public relations efforts.

As reported by the *Los Angeles Times* in August of 2014, the owners of a Northern California slaughterhouse were indicted for ordering employees to process cows with eye cancer stamped as "USDA Condemned." Workers cut the condemned stamps out of the hides and switched the heads with those of healthy cows during meat inspectors' lunch breaks. The USDA initiated a recall of 10 million pounds of such tainted beef already distributed to stores such as Kroger, Food 4 Less and Wal-Mart.

The investigative reporter Eric Schlosser's 2001 book *Fast Food Nation* reveals routine problems in modern slaughterhouses. The typical employees are immigrants without documentation or English proficiency, so that they cannot read posted safety and health notices. Even if they could, slaughterhouse owners speed up the line past the pace where workers can observe procedures for cleanliness. Cutting cows open quickly and without sterilizing the knife in between animals guarantees that meat from a sick cow will contaminate the batch containing hundreds of pounds of hamburger from many other animals. It is also nearly impossible to clean all of the manure from the hides, crusted on from standing in the feedlot. So it is a virtual certainly that the batch of hamburger meat will contain some manure, a cause of *e coli* contamination that can lead to food poisoning.

We all like to imagine that the cows, pigs and chickens we consume lead idyllic lives before they get to the slaughterhouse. We imagine them grazing on green hills, sitting in the sunshine, and leading peaceful lives in a natural environment. But for most animals eventually brought to slaughter such fantasies are far from the truth. A typical commercial feedlot will crowd up to 100,000 cattle at a time onto one square mile where they stand on top of their own manure while they fatten up for market. Their growth is artificially accelerated using antibiotics and growth hormones. Some 80% of antibiotics sold in the U. S. are given to poultry and livestock, mixed with their feed to make them grow faster. And since the antibiotics reduce the risk of infections spreading quickly through the herd, the animals can be kept in relatively unsanitary conditions. A grass-fed cow will take approximately two years to reach market weight, while a feedlot animal will take only 14 months. Only recently has the role of antibiotics in quickly fattening animals become understood. Antibiotics, it turns out, make changes to the bacterium which makes up the microbiome found in the guts of all animals which helps digest carbohydrates. Antibiotics seem to increase the ability to break down carbs. In cattle these drugs cause their metabolism to favor the deposit of protein over fat. Lean muscle weighs more than an equivalent volume of fat so the result is heavier weight gain on the feedlot, commanding higher prices at slaughter.

The dosing promotes antibiotic-resistant strains of bacteria, resulting in salmonella in factory farms. In turn, antibiotic residues in the meat can encourage antibiotic-resistant bacteria in humans, reducing the effectiveness of these drugs in treating human diseases. In addition to the antibiotics, a half-dozen anabolic steroids are given to nearly all animals raised on beef feedlots in the U.S. and Canada. When these animals are slaughtered, measurable levels of hormones remain in the muscle, fat, liver, kidneys and other organ meats. Such residues may be linked to lower sperm counts in boys, and to the development of breast, prostate and colon cancers. As a result of these and other concerns, the European Union, which does not allow the use of hormones in cattle production, has banned the importation of such hormone-treated beef since 1988.

Raw meat and poultry are considered biohazards even by the USDA, which strongly advises consumers to avoid using plates or utensils that have touched raw meat for any other food use, to avoid washing meats and poultry so as not to contaminate sink and counter areas, and to cook such animal products thoroughly. In 1993 Jack in the Box restaurants disregarded Washington State laws requiring burgers to be cooked to at least 155 degrees while promoting "Monster Burger" sandwiches at a discount. The result was widespread e coli contamination from the undercooked meat. Most victims were children under 10 years old. Four children died and 178 other victims sustained permanent injuries including kidney and brain damage. In July of 2000, 60 people were infected with e coli and a 3-year-old girl died due to cross-contamination between meat processing areas and ready-to-eat food preparation areas at Wisconsin Sizzler restaurants. Massive meat recalls occur with regularity in the U. S. Between 1995 and 2000, the USDA enacted 275 recalls for meat products totaling more than 140 million pounds. Of all the recalls completed, less than 30 percent of the contaminated meat was recovered.

Some contamination hazards from commercial meat processing can be indirect. Manure piled up in mountains on cattle feedlots dries out and then blows into adjacent agricultural fields, with the potential to contaminate the crops with *e coli*. Holding ponds of pig manure on hog farms can overflow when it rains, their contents spilling into streams and contaminating groundwater. Other realities of large-scale meat production:

- The total cattle population for the world is approximately 1.3 billion occupying some 24% of the land on the planet.
- Some 70 to 80% of grain produced in the United States is fed to livestock.
- Half the water consumed in the U.S. is used to grow grain for cattle feed.
- A gallon of gasoline is required to produce a pound of grain-fed beef.
- Overall, animal farms use nearly 40 percent of the world's total grain production.
- Hundreds of thousands of acres of tropical forests in Central and South America have been leveled to create grazing land for cattle.

Junk-food chains, including KFC and Pizza Hut, are under attack from major environmental groups in the United States and other developed countries because of their environmental impact. Intensive breeding of livestock and poultry for such restaurants leads to deforestation, land degradation, and contamination of water sources and other natural resources. For every pound of red meat, poultry, eggs, and milk produced, farm fields lose about five pounds of irreplaceable top soil. The water necessary for meat breeding comes to about 190 gallons per animal per day.

--Vandana Shiva, *Stolen Harvest*,
South End Press, 2000, pp. 70-71

Then there is the issue of cattle feed. Cows are vegetarians, suited to eating grass. But on feedlots they are given mostly corn and soybeans for the last few months before slaughter to boost their growth rate and make the meat tenderer, known as "finishing" in the industry. Cornell University researchers found that feeding cattle hay (rather than corn or soybeans) for their last week before slaughter reduces level of *e coli* bacteria in their feces. Since *e coli* live in the cow's intestinal tract, feces escaping during slaughter can contaminate the meat. *(Francisco Diez-Gonzalez, Todd R. Callaway, Menas G. Kizoulis, James B. Russell. "Grain Feeding and the Dissemination of Acid-Resistant Escherichia coli from Cattle" Science, 281 (5383):1666-1668, September 11, 1998).*

Poultry litter is the agriculture industry's term for what gets scooped off the floors of chicken cages and broiler houses, a combination of feces, feathers, and uneaten chicken feed. A typical sample of poultry litter can also contain antibiotics, heavy metals, disease-causing bacteria, and even bits of dead rodents, according to Consumers Union. Aside from the fact that we're feeding our cows chicken crap, this practice is worrisome because the poultry litter can also contain beef protein which is an ingredient in the poultry feed, including ground-up meat and bone meal. That means that cows could be, indirectly, eating *each other*. Meat and bone meal containing infected bovine protein, according to the USDA, is the chief culprit behind the spread of mad cow disease.

Cattle are also administered nitrites, a known carcinogen, to color the meat. Research has linked nitrites to higher rates of colorectal, stomach and pancreatic cancer. Even more nitrites are used in the curing of processed meats such as bacon, ham, lunch meats and hot dogs. Many health and consumer organizations have recommended avoiding such processed meat products altogether as serious health risks. *("The Politics of Meat," Steve Johnson, PBS Frontline)*

Poultry conditions

Conditions in which most poultry in the U. S. are raised are no better, even arguably worse since for the six weeks of their short lives chickens don't even get to see the light of day. Instead they are crammed into huge windowless sheds holding up to 40,000 birds each. Since such numbers make any normal pecking order impossible, the birds relentlessly peck at each other with inevitable injuries and deaths. According to data gathered by People for the Ethical Treatment of Animals, in 2010, just one company, Tyson, "processed" (slaughtered) an average of 42.3 million chickens. In 1925, the average Tyson chicken lived approximately 112 days, weighed around 2.5 pounds at the time of slaughter, and had consumed about 4.7 pounds of grain per pound of its body weight. In 2010, the same chicken lived just 45 days, yet reached an average weight of 5.63 pounds, and consumed only 1.92 pounds of grain per pound. So today's animals live less than half as long, eat half as much and grow more than double the size they did 100 years ago.

As with beef cattle standing in their own manure, chickens are forced to breathe ammonia and particulate matter from feces and feathers all day long. Such conditions cause many to suffer from chronic respiratory diseases, weakened immune systems, bronchitis, and a painful eye condition known as "ammonia burn." And since disease can sweep through a flock rapidly, chickens are given nearly four times the amount of antibiotics as human beings or cattle in the United States. Such dosing leads to antibiotic-resistant bacteria; a 2006 study by *Consumer Reports* found that 83 percent of grocery market chickens it tested were infected with either campylobacter or salmonella bacteria or both. That is why it is routine for consumer advice organizations, especially around Thanksgiving time, to warn people to avoid using any utensils coming in contact with the raw poultry for any other food preparation.

When it comes to what the factory-farmed chickens are fed, the US Food and Drug Administration wisely banned the practice of feeding the remains of dead cows to living ones back in 1997 in order to help prevent mad cow disease. However, the FDA has not prohibited feeding cattle remains to chickens and other poultry, nor does it currently prohibit feeding poultry litter to cattle, which means that the risk of mad cow disease is reintroduced in this legal but worrisome (and disgusting) exchange loop. Certainly chickens are not designed by nature to eat beef, and cows are vegetarian animals, designed to eat grass.

Besides that risk, arsenic has routinely been fed to poultry (and sometimes hogs) because it reduces infections and turns the flesh an appetizing shade of pink. Chickens are sometimes fed coffee pulp and green tea powder to keep them awake so that they can spend more time eating. Then they are given does of Benadryl to calm them down. They are also administered nitrites, a known carcinogen, to color the meat. As noted above, research has linked nitrites to higher rates of colorectal, stomach and pancreatic cancer.

Eggs

When it comes to egg-laying "battery hens," their year of life is spent crammed into a small wire cage with up to nine other hens in a shed holding up to 125,000 other tormented birds. In a natural environment hens roam, scratch, forage and enjoy dust baths with flock mates, but all those normal activities are denied by the battery environment. Hens are debeaked with a hot machine blade so that they cannot peck at each other and cause damage. This is done at one day old and again at seven weeks since the beak will often grow back. Debeaking affects the hen's ability to properly eat, drink and preen.

Egg-laying hens are dosed with antibiotics not just to prevent disease due to crowded confinement, but to boost egg production. While wild hens might lay two clutches of a dozen eggs per year, battery hens are chemically manipulated to produce 250. Such abnormal production drains too much calcium from hens' bones to form the egg shells, resulting in osteoporosis than can eventually paralyze them so that they die of hunger and thirst lying within inches of their water and food. Many reproductive maladies afflict birds deprived of normal exercise and forced to lay abnormally large numbers of eggs. When hens' oviducts become infested with salmonella, the bacteria enter the forming egg and can cause food poisoning for consumers. Toxic ammonia from decomposing uric acid in manure pits beneath the cage, besides burning the birds' eyes and respiratory systems, will also be absorbed into the eggs. So one lesson here is that, even if people have no sympathy for the suffering of the birds, the conditions under which they live in effect poison and nutritionally degrade the very product that all of these unnatural arrangements are made to produce. Salmonella contamination is one typical outcome from such conditions. In 2010 over half a billion eggs were recalled for salmonella contamination.

Consumers can try the option of buying "free-range" or "cage-free" "organic" eggs. Free-range or cage-free means chickens are given access to the outdoors at least 51% of the time. Of course access is not a guarantee of how much time a hen will actually spend outdoors, and they can still live in crowded henhouses. And unfortunately there is no clear evidence that such practice decreases salmonella risk in the eggs. As reported by CNN (August 26, 2010), "no matter how carefully eggs are produced and handled, or regulated, it is impossible to guarantee that a raw egg is free of salmonella or other harmful bacteria." If eggs are labeled organic hens must be given feed containing no toxic pesticides, herbicides, or fungicides and no GMOs or slaughterhouse by-products. While this seems promising, the best indicator of quality eggs will be those from hens in the least crowded facilities—the opposite of conditions for commercial battery hens.

Pigs

About 100 million pigs are raised each year for in the U. S. Most are slaughtered by the age of six months. To give an idea of the scale of factory farming, Kansas regulators in 2014 approved a massive expansion at a Seaboard Foods' hog farm, permitting up to 396,000 pigs. The Seaboard operation will generate twice as much waste as the city of Wichita, and will tax the area's already diminished water supply which is dependent on the depleted Ogallala Aquifer underlying it.

Some infectious hazards are particularly associated with hog farming. *Yersinia enterocolitica* is a bacterium that is found in 69 percent of tested pork samples. It can cause fever, diarrhea and abdominal pain, infecting 100,000 Americans a year, especially children. Intensive confinement of pigs in factory farms also incubated the highly infectious H1N1 virus that led to a global pandemic of "swine flu" in 2009. According to the Institute for Southern Studies, drinking water contaminated with nitrates from hog farm runoff increases the risk of blue baby syndrome, which can be fatal. High levels of nitrates in drinking water near hog farms have also been linked to spontaneous abortions.

The state of Iowa experienced 51 manure spills and 25 air-quality violations due to hog farming in 2013. The animal waste accumulated in holding pools often overflows into local streams and groundwater sources. The mortality rate on hog farms (during the time when the animals are being raised for slaughter) averages 10 percent. A recent rash of PED (Porcine Epidemic Diarrhea) in North Carolina killed millions of pigs and their corpses, and as is typical, their corpses were buried in shallow mass graves, a practice that can transmit bacteria and pathogens to drinking water supplies and recreational waters.

For those who might be moved by considerations of animal cruelty, pigs on factory farms are confined to small concrete pens, without bedding or soil or hay for rooting. Yet pigs are highly intelligent animals who naturally lead social lives of a complexity approaching that of primates. The stress of being deprived of normal social interaction causes some pigs to bite the tails off of other pigs. Factory farm operators respond by cutting off their tails. They make other modifications to the animals to streamline their industrial operation: male piglets have their testicles cut out of their scrotums, many of their teeth clipped in half, and their ears mutilated, all without any pain relief. They are crammed into pens and given almost no room to move, because, in the economics of the pork industry, overcrowding pigs pays.

Sows are artificially inseminated and confined for the entire length of their pregnancies in "gestation crates," cages just 2 feet wide, too small for them to even turn around or lie down comfortably. After three or four years of continuous pregnancies under conditions of loneliness and deprivation the sows' bodies are exhausted and they are shipped off to slaughter. Gestation and farrowing crates are viewed by many animal experts as so barbaric that they have been banned in several U.S. states as well in the U.K. and Sweden.

The good news is that there are now readily available alternatives on the market to replace bacon, bacon bits, and sausages. There are also chicken substitutes, the famous Tofurkey and related products, vegetable-derived deli slices, veggie hot dogs, and a variety of veggie burgers. As more Americans have opted out of eating meat, food companies large and small have innovated to meet demand for meat substitutes in great variety.

Fish

It would be consoling to think that fish might serve as a reasonable alternative to eating red meat, pigs, or poultry. Yet unfortunately there are problems connected to this important world protein source. Fish is lower in fat than red meat and higher in healthful omega-3 fatty acids. But over many years we have polluted our oceans with mercury, plastics and chemicals. Fish high up on the food chain, referred to as top predators, such as king mackerel, shark, and swordfish, are consistently high in mercury. Other fish, including canned light tuna, can also be high in that metal. Women who are pregnant or nursing or who may become pregnant and young children are particularly at risk from mercury. A U.S. Environmental Protection Agency (EPA) analysis released in 2004 indicated that about 630,000 of the 4 million children born annually in the U.S. are at risk of impaired motor function, learning capacity, memory, and vision due to high levels of mercury in their bloodstreams. The mercury hazard is clear enough that consumer organizations advise people to consume no more than 3 ounces of fish for children or six ounces for adults *per week.*

Industrial and municipal wastes and agricultural chemicals flushed into the world's waters are absorbed by the fish which live there. Big fish, such as tuna and salmon, eat smaller fish. The bigger the fish, the greater the potential accumulation of toxic chemicals in their bodies. Pollutants that concentrate in fish include pesticides; polychlorinated biphenyls (PCBs); toxic metals such as lead, cadmium, chromium, and arsenic; dioxins; and radioactive substances such as strontium 90. Because of biological magnification as they move up the food chain, pollutants can reach levels as high as 9 million times that of the water in which they live. Nursing infants consume half of their mother's load of PCBs, dioxin, DDT, and other toxic chemicals. These toxins have been linked to cancers, nervous system disorders, fetal damage, and many other serious health effects. Besides the problems of mercury, chemicals and radioactive wastes, in a six-month investigation, Consumers Union found that nearly half the fish tested from markets in New York City, Chicago, and Santa Cruz, California were contaminated by bacteria from human or nonhuman feces. In addition, fish often contain disease-causing worms and parasites.

In the face of these problems largely related to pollution, people might think that the safer bet is to go with "farmed" fish. Yet here we find a familiar scenario to the production of factory-farmed meat. In the U. S., in order to maximize profit, most "farmed" trout, salmon, catfish, and other fish are raised in the same sort of intensive crowding found in commercial chicken and pig operations. Like those industries, fish "farming" involves large-scale, highly mechanized production. Thousands of fish are crammed into ponds, troughs, or sea-floating cages, so that fish farmers can raise the greatest possible number of fish per cubic foot of water. In most cases, each fish is allotted a space scarcely larger than its body. Farmed fish are fed pellets designed for unnaturally rapid weight gain. Under these abnormal intensely crowded conditions, fish suffer from stress, infections, parasites, oxygen depletion, and gas bubble disease (similar to "the bends" in humans). In an effort to prevent the spread of disease among the fish, producers give them large amounts of antibiotics.

Then there are environmental considerations. Fish "farming" depletes natural resources. It requires as much as twenty calories of fossil-fuel energy to produce one calorie of energy from fish. Fish grown in artificial ponds require vast amounts of water to replenish oxygen and remove wastes. Raising one ton of fish for slaughter requires eight tons of water. Producing one pound of flesh from captive fish requires three to four pounds of flesh from wild fish, so eating farmed fish decimates populations of free-living fish. Accumulated wastes from fish farms pollute the local marine environment and spread illnesses. When farmed fish, laden with antibiotics, escape and breed with free-living fish, aquatic ecosystems may be thrown out of balance because of the mating of wild and farmed fish. Escaped fish raised in intensive confinement may spread disease to free populations of fish.

Even setting aside the issue of contamination from pollutants, today's fishing practices also wreak havoc on our environment. Modern commercial trawlers the size of a football field, using sonar technology to locate fish and giant nets sometimes miles long, scoop up everything in their path. They can net 800,000 pounds of fish in just one sweep. Trawling scrapes up ocean bottoms and destroys coral reefs which are crucial to the nourishment of aquatic life. Half of the fish and other sea creatures caught through commercial fishing are fed to animals raised for food, including the "farmed" fish. Each year, about 30 million tons of aquatic animals, some on endangered species lists, maimed, dying, or already dead, are simply tossed back into the ocean.

The global fishing fleet is two to three times larger than what the oceans can sustainably support. Due to such industrial fishing the number of large predatory fish has dramatically declined over the last 50 years. About 80 percent of all the top predatory fish are gone from coastal areas of the North Pacific and North Atlantic. As these important fish are lost they are replaced by smaller, faster-growing species like plankton-feeding fish and shellfish, leading to potentially irreversible shifts in entire ocean ecosystems. 63 percent of global fish stocks are now considered overfished. The idea that fish can magically replace themselves is unrealistic. An instructive example is Newfoundland in Canada where for centuries the stock of cod in the Grand Banks seemed inexhaustible. Yet by 1992 that cod fishery collapsed, causing 40,000 people to lose their jobs, including 10,000 fishermen.

While it is less common to have compassion for the lives of fish compared to those of animals, it is unlikely that fish are beyond suffering. When fish are hauled up from a considerable depth, the sudden change in pressure on their bodies causes painful decompression that often causes their gills to collapse and their eyes to pop out. As soon as fish are removed from water, they begin to suffocate. We have already considered the overcrowding and artificial means of fish farms; it is unlikely that people would subject their pet fish that they keep at home in bowls and aquariums to such conditions.

Obviously super-trawling for fish and fish farming are driven by consumer demand, so the more people who turn to alternative vegetarian foods instead of consuming fish, the less damage will be done to our already-damaged marine ecosystems. So far as the benefits of omega-3 fatty acids, the most cursory research will show that there is actually little scientific evidence for their possible benefits. And there are healthier plant-based sources of these acids, especially from flax seeds, canola, soybean, walnuts, tofu, pumpkin, and wheat germ. Further, these plant foods provide health-promoting fiber and antioxidants. And they don't contain the toxic heavy metals and carcinogens found in fish flesh.

It must be added that food horror stories don't stop with an overview of animals processed for meat. The pursuit of profit above all else leads to abuses and danger for consumers well beyond the animal protein arena. Dairy products will be considered in a separate chapter of this book. Just to pick a few out of many unfortunate examples of food industry abuses, some decades ago when "diet" and "high fiber" breads hit the market, parent company ITT Continental Bakeries eventually admitted that the ingredient they used for low-calorie fiber in Profile and Fresh Horizons bread was sawdust. In 1979 the Federal Trade Commission charged ITT Continental Baking Company with false and misleading advertising because it had not disclosed that the alpha cellulose in its bread Fresh Horizons came from wood pulp. Other breads containing wood pulp included Roman Meal and more. The sawdust is processed powder or pulp from virgin wood, and the practice has not been discontinued, but has actually increased in recent years.

Since the ingredient is not toxic, the FDA says it's okay to use in food. The food industry and FDA classify wood cellulose as fiber. The only limit on wood cellulose fillers is 3.5% in meat. All other foods have no limits for adding wood cellulose. From the industry point of view, cellulose adds to shelf life, and manufacturers can promote their products as "lower fat, higher fiber." Above all, it amounts to cheap filler that can make foods taste creamier without as much fat. It keeps shredded cheese from lumping together.

Wood cellulose is not toxic. But it's not food either. Our enzymes cannot digest cellulose. Cellulose in the ingredients list is a giveaway. Wood-derived cellulose is used by various companies in waffles, pancakes, snack bars, syrups, muffins, low-fat ice cream, sour cream, yogurt, non-dairy creamers, crackers, pizza crusts, muffins, scrambled eggs, mashed potato mixes, breakfast cereals, cake mixes, BBQ sauce, macaroni & cheese, nacho chips, pasta sauces, hot cocoa mixes, and even cheesecake. The only defense is to read labels carefully and avoid heavily processed foods.

Another instructive tale concerns 15-year-old high school student Sara Kavanagh from Mississippi who noticed that one of the listed ingredients in Gatorade was brominated vegetable oil or BVO. BVO is part of the same chemical family as flame-retardants like polybrominated diphenyl ether (PBDE). The beverage industry uses it to help citrus-flavored soft drinks keep a uniform color in the bottles. The chemical was banned in Japan and Europe but added to about 10 percent of soda in Northern America since the 1930s.

Side effects of BVO include skin rashes, severe acne, fatigue, loss of appetite, abdominal pain, metallic taste, and cardiac arrhythmias. In one case a man who consumed two to four liters of a soda containing BVO on a daily basis experienced memory loss, tremors, fatigue, loss of muscle coordination, headache, and ptosis or drooping of the right eyelid. Over the two months it took to correctly diagnose the problem, the patient also lost the ability to walk. He needed dialysis as part of his treatment but eventually recovered. Bromines are also common endocrine disruptors, and if you are exposed to a lot of bromine, your body will not hold on to the iodine that it needs. Iodine affects every tissue in your body, not just your thyroid. Approximately 10% of Americans suffer from hypothyroidism or lowered metabolism.

Sarah Kavanagh, the high school student, started an online petition to remove this dangerous ingredient from Gatorade. When her petition quickly gathered over 200,000 signatures, parent company Pepsico agreed to remove

BVO, though it temporarily left it in Mountain Dew and other drinks. Other companies such as Coca-Cola also used the ingredient. Finally in May of 2014, Coca-Cola and PepsiCo said they would remove BVO from all of their products.

BVO was "generally recognized as safe" by the FDA when first used as an additive decades ago. But in 1970 it was removed from the GRAS list. Nevertheless it was still permitted in limited amounts. Sarah observed that since BVO had been banned for beverage use in Europe and Japan, yet Pepsico's drinks were still sold in those countries, they must clearly have devised an alternative formula. Some lessons here are that our FDA cannot be trusted to always protect consumers against dangerous ingredients. Also, one has to wonder why it took a 15-year-old girl to call these giant corporations on their hazardous and unnecessary practices rather than the very agencies we created and pay for with taxpayer dollars to protect us. Undoubtedly the use of BVO proved cheaper than the alternative, and so in the absence of any firm regulations against their use, food companies knowingly went ahead with the marketing of beverages that pose a health risk to consumers.

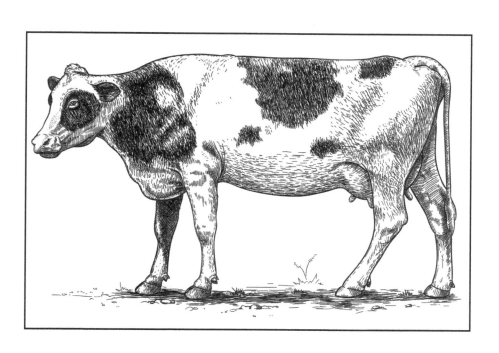

Dairy Products

"We are the only animal who continues to drink milk after weaning... Pasteurized milk is as deadly as meat, yet so many vegetarians take this path of slow suicide."
                    --Viktoras Kulvinskas, *Survival into the 21ˢᵗ Century*

Abandoning meat-eating is a big step toward vegetarianism. After a typical American childhood, it involves a break with tradition and habit that can be difficult even when armed with the great body of information now available about the harm and risks to health that come with consuming animal flesh, particularly due to the ways animals are processed for food. Yet how many 'lacto-ovo' vegetarians go on to eat as vegans, abandoning as well the consumption of eggs and dairy products? The propaganda and advertising from organizations such as the National Dairy Council have been so effective in convincing people that these foods are irreplaceable in the diet that such an attitude has been absorbed into American culture. If baseball, apple pie and ice cream are proverbially at the core of what it means to be American, who is going to give up ice cream? Most never think to question this national habit or learn about the actual contents of dairy foods and their potential effects on health. (Eggs have already been discussed in detail in the Food Horror Stories chapter).

Dairy consumption has played an increasing role in the American diet over the last 100 years. As a point of reference, over the course of the 20ᵗʰ century Americans increased their meat consumption from about 120 pounds each to about 222 pounds per year. When it comes to dairy, Americans increased their consumption from about 294 pounds per year each to a whopping 605 pounds! Worth mentioning is that they also more than tripled their intake of refined sugar from 40 to 147 pounds This information comes from the worthwhile documentary *Forks Over Knives*, directed by Lee Fulkerson.

Part of the increase in dairy consumption was due to the development of refrigeration and freezing so that products could be transported further and stored longer at home before spoiling. Today our markets present a parade of ice cream, yogurt, frozen yogurt, cottage cheese, sour cream, whipping cream, milk in many varieties of fat contents and flavors, condensed milk, evaporated milk, butter, cheese, cream cheese and more. What all this boils down to are many ways to deliver to consumers the commercial product of dairy foods in multiple guises. I keep a copy of a book published and distributed free to grade-school children purporting to give the "History of the World" in just a few pages. Placed right up there with the discovery of fire and the development of agriculture in this version of human history is the domestication of animals for dairy products! And who published this children's guide? The National Dairy Council.

The propaganda continues on into adulthood with ad campaigns such as the "Got Milk?" series depicting adult athletes and celebrities wearing milk mustaches and claiming (or being paid to claim) that they owe their health and strength partly to drinking milk. Posters of these milk mustache-wearing actors, sports figures, musicians, and models are sent to 60,000 U.S. elementary schools and 45,000 middle and high schools; shades of the "History of the World" campaign! The industry even tried marketing dairy products as helpful for weight loss until the Federal Trade Commission's Bureau of Consumer Protection directed milk marketers to stop their weight-loss campaign since any such claim required further research to provide stronger evidence of any association between dairy consumption and weight loss.

> Healthcare professionals, unless subsidized by the dairy industry, seldom recommend milk because of its cholesterol, fat, calories, allergens and impurities and its possible links to rBGH (recombinant bovine growth hormone) since milk made with the cow milk enhancer has never been labeled. Benjamin Spock, the famous baby boom-era pediatrician, recommended no milk for children after age two to reduce their risks of heart disease, obesity, high blood pressure, diabetes, and diet-related cancers. In a 2001 USDA expert panel report panelists found whole milk could increase the

risk of prostate cancer and heart disease and ads should include such warnings.

("Got Propaganda?" by Martha Rosenberg;
http://www.alternet.org/story/154443, March 12, 2012)

So what are the problems with milk?

Cow's milk is suited to the nutritional needs of calves, which have four stomachs and gain hundreds of pounds over a matter of months, so that some weigh more than 1,000 pounds by the time they are two years old. No other mammals drink milk after weaning in infancy, and humans are definitely the only species that drinks another species' milk. Most people begin to produce less lactase, the enzyme that helps with the digestion of milk, when they are as young as two years old. Low levels of that enzyme can lead to lactose intolerance. Millions of Americans are in fact lactose intolerant, including an estimated 90 percent of Asian-Americans and 75 percent of Native- and African-Americans. Lactase intolerance can cause bloating, gas, cramps, vomiting, headaches, rashes, and asthma.

Cows' milk, both regular and 'organic,' contains 59 active hormones, scores of allergens, fat and cholesterol. Most cows' milk also contains herbicides, pesticides, dioxins up to 200 times the safe levels, as many as 52 powerful antibiotics, blood, pus, feces, bacteria and viruses. It can also contain detergent residues from the cleaning of the milk machines. These contents will gain concentration in other forms of dairy. Each bite of hard cheese has *ten times* whatever was in that sip of milk, because it takes ten pounds of milk to make one pound of cheese. Each bite of ice cream has 12 times, and every swipe of butter has 21 times whatever is contained in the fat molecules in a sip of milk.

Again, as with animals raised for meat, we must revise our childhood images of happy cows grazing on green hillsides and face up to the reality of modern milk processing. After their calves are taken away from them, mother cows are hooked up, several times a day, to milking machines which were developed on a commercial basis in the 1970s. These cows are genetically manipulated, artificially inseminated, and often drugged to force them to produce about four and a half times as much milk as they naturally would to feed their calves.

There are more than 9 million cows on U.S. dairy farms, which is actually fewer than there were in 1950. Yet milk production has continued to increase, from 116 billion pounds of milk per year in 1950 to 185 billion pounds in 2007. Normally, these animals would produce only enough milk to meet the needs of their calves, about 6,000 pounds per year, but with genetic manipulation and the use of antibiotics and hormones production has been boosted to more than 20,000 pounds of milk each year. Cows are also fed unnatural, high-protein diets including dead chickens, pigs, and other animals since their natural diet of grass would not provide the nutrients that they need to produce such massive amounts of milk.

The bovine growth hormone BGH is used widely in the U.S. even though is has been banned in Europe and Canada because of concerns over human health and animal welfare. The use of BGH contributes to a painful inflammation of the udder known as "mastitis" which according to the industry's own figures afflicts between 30 and 50 percent of dairy cows. There are about 150 bacteria that can cause the disease, one of which is *E. coli*. The infected cows shed somatic cells, or what in humans would be called pus, into the milk. While a healthy somatic cell count (SCC) would be 100,000 cells per milliliter, the USDA permits up to seven times that amount. Elevated SCC is associated with using automatic milking machines. The European Union and Canada limit the SCC to 400,000 pus cells per milliliter. It is not uncommon for blood to get into the milk from the inflamed udders of cows suffering from mastitis. In routine industry testing of milk batches with as much as 1% blood content it is difficult to detect discoloration. So in effect milk can also contain significant amounts of cows' blood.

According to the American Gastroenterological Association, cow's milk is the number one cause of food allergies among infants and children. A U.K. study showed that people who suffered from irregular heartbeats, asthma, headaches, fatigue, and digestive problems showed marked and often complete improvements in their health after cutting milk from their diets (Carrell, S. "Milk causes serious illness for 7M Britons." *The Independent*, June 22, 2003). A study at Great Ormond Street Children's Hospital in London found that the food most likely to trigger a migraine was cow's milk. The conclusion is that the possibility of cow's milk allergy or intolerance should be considered in all cases of migraine.

The proteins in dairy can cause allergies. The Mayo Clinic reports that casein and whey, the two main proteins in cow's milk, are identified by our immune systems as harmful, triggering the production of antibodies that in turn set off a range of allergic reactions whenever your body comes in contact with those proteins.

For those concerned about dietary cholesterol, it is worth noting that the cholesterol content of those three glasses of milk is equal to what one would get from 53 slices of bacon. The saturated fats in dairy can increase risk of heart disease and other health problems.

For those concerned about animal welfare, one of the ingredients used for cheese-making is rennet, a complex of enzymes found in the stomach of baby mammals that allows them to process mother's milk. In cheese-making rennet helps separate curds and whey and facilitates coagulation. Animal rennet comes from the stomach of newborn calves, lambs, and kids (baby goats). Vegetable rennet, made from plant sources, is an alternative, and will be listed on the label, though it may also be made from genetically modified soybeans. Since genetically engineered rennet doesn't have to be labeled, people concerned about GMOs will want to avoid it. Clearly buying or making non-dairy cheese avoids all of the issues raised here.

Dr. Ganmaa Davaasambuu, working at the Harvard School of Public Health and citing detailed research studies, found that milk and cheese consumption are strongly correlated to the incidence of hormone-dependent cancer, particularly breast cancer, prostate cancer, and testicular cancer among men ages 20 to 39. Rates were highest in places like Switzerland and Denmark, where cheese is a national food.

Milk contains 59 different bioactive hormones that might be linked to early onset of puberty. In 1973 in Michigan, cattle were accidentally fed grain contaminated with an estrogen-mimicking chemical, the flame retardant PBB. The daughters born to the pregnant women who ate the PBB-laced meat and drank the PBB-laced milk started menstruating significantly earlier than their peers.

Dairy consumption has been linked to the onset of Type 1 diabetes. This finding has been tracked across many countries. Japanese children, who have the lowest milk consumption, have $1/36^{th}$ the incidence of Type-1 diabetes compared to children from Finland, with the highest consumption of milk. (T. Colin Campbell, *The China Study*).

80% of the protein in milk is casein, which is used to make commercial glues like the kind kids use in school. You can dial up YouTube videos that show how to make glue from milk on your stovetop using vinegar and baking soda. The protein casein in dairy products can create serious problems just like the protein gluten in some grains like wheat. They can trigger an autoimmune response and/or mimic endorphins to cause changes in perception, mood, and behavior. Those pursuing a "gluten-free" diet would do well to take this into consideration.

A pioneer of the natural health movement in America, Dr. Paavo Airola, reported that pasteurization and homogenization, part of the routine processing of commercial milk, actually degrade raw milk.

> Pasteurization (heating mike to 165 degrees for 20 seconds) destroys significant levels of vitamin C present in raw milk and reduces the level of B-complex vitamins...Calcium levels are reduced by a leaching that happens in milk handling. The enzymes destroyed would aid milk absorption. Pasteurization also neutralized an antibody which would otherwise retard bacterial growth. Homogenization, the permanent blending of milk and cream for commercial milk, may render cream fats so small that they pass directly into the bloodstream without digestion, increasing serum fat levels.
> (Airola, *Are You Confused.* Phoenix: Health Plus, 1987)

A persistent belief is that we need cows' milk for calcium, which is reinforced by industry advertising. The suggestion is that milk builds strong bones. Yet it is worth reflecting that the cows themselves, who are naturally vegetarians, get all the calcium they need for strong bones from plants, which also provide large amounts of magnesium needed for the absorption of calcium. Milk itself has only enough magnesium to aid absorption of around 11% of its calcium content.

> Clinical research shows that dairy products have little or no benefit for bones. A 2005 review published in *Pediatrics* showed that milk consumption does not improve bone integrity in children. In a more recent study, researchers tracked the diets,

physical activity, and stress fracture incidences of adolescent girls for seven years, and concluded that dairy products and calcium do not prevent stress fractures in adolescent girls. Similarly, the Harvard Nurses' Health Study, which followed more than 72,000 women for 18 years, showed no protective effect of increased milk consumption on fracture risk.

(Physicians Committee on Responsible Medicine; http://www.pcrm. org/health/diets/vegdiets/health-concerns-about-dairy-products)

Leafy greens provide plenty of absorbable calcium, as do soy milk and soybeans, tofu, broccoli, collards, kale, mustard greens, okra and more.

Dairy cows hardly lead natural lives. A cow's natural lifespan is about 25 years, but cows used by the dairy industry are killed after only four or five years. An industry study reports that by the time they are killed, nearly 40 percent of dairy cows are lame because of the intensive confinement, the filth, and the strain of being almost constantly pregnant and giving milk. Dairy cows' bodies are turned into soup, pet food, or low-grade hamburger meat (beef for fast food) because their bodies are too "spent" to be used for anything else.

Environmental Destruction

Large dairy farms have an enormously detrimental effect on the environment. In California, America's top milk-producing state, manure from dairy farms has poisoned hundreds of square miles of groundwater, rivers, and streams. Each of the more than one million cows on the state's dairy farms excretes 18 gallons of manure daily, much of which ends up in waterways and drinking water. The Environmental Protection Agency reports that agricultural runoff is the primary cause of polluted lakes, streams, and rivers in the U. S. The dairy industry is also one of the primary sources of smog-forming pollutants in California; a single cow emits more of these harmful gasses than a car does. In addition, two-thirds of all agricultural land in the U.S. is used to raise animals for food or to grow grain to feed them. Each cow raised by the dairy industry consumes as much as 40 gallons of water per day, which is quite significant in states like California which are prone to severe draughts.

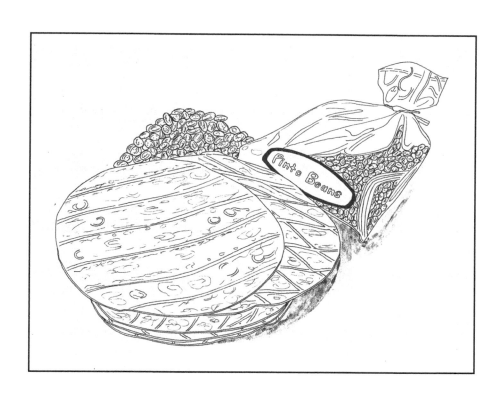

On Protein

Most Americans have come to believe that the more protein they get the better. This notion leads to the religion of the 32-ounce steak as a sign of success, good nourishment and even masculinity! Yet people can get too much protein, which has been linked to a number of health problems, including kidney stones and osteoporosis. Unlike fats and carbohydrates, protein can't be stored by the human body. Any consumed protein that exceeds the amount that can be used on a given day is broken down and excreted. After someone eats concentrated protein, such as a salmon steak, meat or dairy cheese, the body must cleanse the blood of protein wastes, such as urea, ammonia, and amino acid fragments. Animal protein is high in sulfur-containing amino acids, which are metabolized into sulfuric acid. This condition is referred to as "increased potential renal acid load resulting from a high protein" intake by the National Institutes of Health. Since cleansing requires calcium, the excess protein, excreted through the urine, puts a strain on the kidneys, causing them to compensate by leaching calcium from the bones. Continued year after year, such calcium loss may result in thin bones that easily fracture: osteoporosis, a condition that affects 15 million Americans. Due to lower acid production, vegetable protein generally causes much less calcium loss.

The Johns Hopkins Medicine website suggests that lack of acid-neutralizing foods, specifically fruits and vegetables, may exacerbate calcium loss. It's very difficult not to get enough calories from protein when you eat a healthy diet; protein deficiency (also known as 'kwashiorkor') is rare in the U.S. and is usually only a problem for people who live in famine-stricken countries. But eating too much animal protein has been linked to the development of endometrial, pancreatic, and prostate cancer. Meat-based protein is also high in saturated fat, which can increase the risk of stroke, coronary heart disease, diabetes and some types of cancer. Worldwide, cultures which eat less animal-protein, including Asian nations, have fewer hip-fractures (a hallmark sign of osteoporosis) than cultures that do eat lots of animal-protein like the USA and UK.

B. J. Abelow et al.: Hip Fracture and Animal Protein

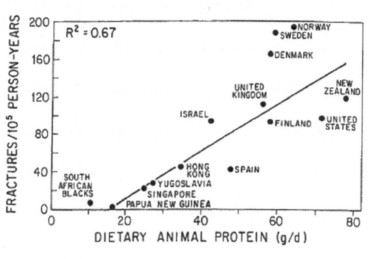

(Calcified Tissue International (1992) 50:14 – 18)

The ingredients of protein are amino acids, which are classified into three groups:

Essential amino acids cannot be made by the body, and must be supplied by food. They do not need to be eaten at one meal, or even on the same day. Basic balance in the diet is more important.

Nonessential amino acids are made by the body from essential amino acids or in the normal breakdown of proteins.

Conditional amino acids are needed in times of illness and stress.

Many Americans take in more protein than they need. The FDA recommends a daily protein intake of 50 grams for a 2,000-calorie diet, which includes built-in extra grams for 'insurance.' Yet the National Health and Nutrition Examination survey found that the average American male consumes over 100 grams of protein per day, twice the RDA, and the average female eats about 70 grams.

Many plants deliver quality protein, as can be noted from this brief sampling on the chart reproduced here (from Vegan Weight Watchers website):

Item	Quantity	Protein	P+
Almonds	15 nuts	3.93 g	3 P+
Asparagus	1 cup	4.32 g	0 P+
Banana	1 large	1.48 g	0 P+
Beans, black	½ cup	7.62 g	2 P+
Blueberries	1 cup	1.1 g	0 P+
Broccoli, cooked	1 cup	3.71 g	0 P+
Brown rice	1 cup	5.03 g	5 P+
Cantelope	¼ large	1.79 g	0 P+
Cauliflower	1 cup	2.27 g	0 P+
Hemp Protein Powder	1 scoop	11g	2 P+
Lentils	1 cup	8.93 g	2 P+
Pea Protein Powder	1 scoop	15g	3 P+
Quinoa	1 cup	7.42 g	5 P+
Walnuts	14 halves	3.04 g	4 P+
Whole wheat pasta	1 cup	7.46 g	4 P+

Greens, legumes, potatoes, nuts and seeds, and grains all deliver protein in varying amounts. So do vegetarian supplements such as chlorella, spirulina, wheatgrass, and hemp powder which are covered in a separate chapter of this book. Soybeans deliver particularly useful protein, as noted by the American Cancer Society:

> Soybean products are promoted for their protective properties against breast, prostate, colon, and lung cancer. The effects of soy are thought by some to be due to substances called isoflavones, sometimes called plant estrogens because they mimic, though weakly, estrogen that is produced in humans and animals. Genistein, daidzein, and glycitein are isoflavones that are present in small amounts in other foods but are most abundant in soy. As a protein source, soybean products are promoted as a healthier alternative to meat and as an aid to weight loss. Soy products are also used to lower cholesterol and blood pressure, and to relieve symptoms of menopause and osteoporosis. Soy protein in a diet low in saturated fat

and cholesterol is also promoted as a method to help reduce the risk of heart disease.

(ACS Guidelines on Nutrition and Physical Activity
for Cancer Prevention; www.cancer.org)

Most plants contain all the essential amino acids, but in varying concentrations. Eating a variety of plant foods forms a complete protein profile and also provides a healthy dose of fiber -- which helps lower cholesterol, promotes regular bowel movements, regulates blood sugar and helps us feel full. Plant-based proteins don't have any saturated fat, and most are lower in calories than the animal protein alternatives. Most plants contain all the essential amino acids, but in varying concentrations.

You ensure you are getting adequate protein you need not keep some chart or load your plate at each meal with perfectly balanced complete protein foods. Your body will do the homework. So long as over the day, the week, or even the month you get a variety of protein, the body will store the excess of one or more amino acids in the liver and other body cells. If one day you get insufficient lysine, the liver will compensate by releasing stored lysine in the bloodstream to provide all essential amino acids for building cells, enzymes and hormones and for other protein functions.

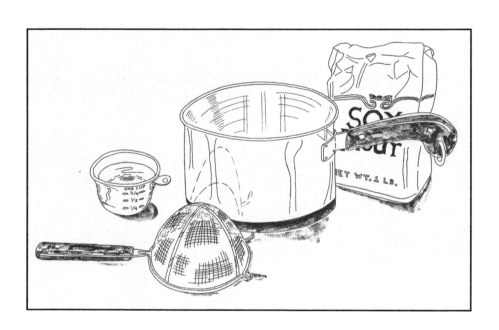

Soymilk and Other Non-Dairy Milks

When discussing soy products we must first take up the matter of whether soy is harmful, as some recent health rumors have suggested. Soy contains *isoflavones* which have the ability to bind to estrogen receptors and can affect the thyroid hormone, particularly if someone has iodine deficiency. But unless you have thyroid issues or are allergic to soy, two servings per day are perfectly safe.

There is another concern that soy could cause feminizing characteristics in men, based upon two case studies, in which the men were consuming 12 to 14 servings of soy a day, a very high intake. Another study used much higher amounts of isoflavones, yet found no problems for most men.

Another issue is *hexane*, a volatile solvent used, with Food and Drug Administration (FDA) approval, to extract oil from soybeans, nuts and olives. Most soy protein ingredients listed on labels as soy protein isolate, soy protein concentrate or textured vegetable protein, undergo hexane processing. According to the Soyfoods Association of North America, hexane is used only in the initial steps of soy processing, and virtually all of it is eliminated by the time soy ingredients are put into soy burgers and other products.

Soy foods made from whole soybeans such as tofu, tempeh, soy milk, and soy yogurt do not typically undergo hexane processing and are generally healthier for you than the extracted isolates. While there is no evidence that the amounts of hexane typically found in soy foods are harmful to consumers, if you want to avoid hexane-treated soy foods, choose products labeled "100% organic" with the USDA seal, since hexane is banned in organic food production. Expeller-pressing and cold-pressing are methods to extract oils that do not involve solvents, so soy and other vegetable oils produced in this manner are also hexane-free. And there are companies that make alternative meats without using hexane, such as Tofurky and Field Roast.

So far as any connection between soy and breast cancer, international studies associate soy with a lower risk for breast cancer or no association, particularly in countries with relatively high soy intake such as China and Japan. Marji McCullough, ScD, RD of the American Cancer Society concurs that there is no evidence of adverse effects of soy foods on breast cancer prognosis. In addition to reducing the risk for breast cancer, soy provides benefits for improving cognition, preventing prostate cancer, lowering LDL cholesterol, and improving menopausal symptoms.

The dairy industry, losing market share to an increasing number of health-conscious Americans, has tried to preserve market share against products such as soy, almond, rice and coconut milks. The National Milk Producers Federation petitioned the FDA to ban words like "milk" and "cheese" from any products that aren't made from dairy milk. Their marketing campaigns try to suggest that dairy is superior nutritionally to the alternative products. But as reported by *Mother Jones* magazine,

> Actually, soy milk and dairy aren't that different nutritionally, except for that milk is fattier. For example, a cup of Trader Joe's vanilla soy milk has 30 less calories than a cup of 2% milk. A cup of soy milk has 0% of your daily saturated fat, while milk has 15%. Dairy does have twice the protein as soy milk, but soy milk has 10% more calcium.
> (*Jen Quraishi, http://www.motherjones.com/blue-marble/2010/04/ dairy-lobby-tries-ban-soy-milk, April 29, 2010*)

So the bottom line is that consumers can choose alternatives to dairy with confidence. While soy milk used to be something found only in health food stores and Chinatowns, now it has become a supermarket staple. It is sold in a variety of flavors including vanilla, chocolate and strawberry, in light or regular versions, and both sweetened and unsweetened. And as mentioned before, there are also now widely available almond, oat, rice, coconut, flax and hempseed milks. In fact you can also make milk out of cashews, sunflower seeds and other seeds and nuts using the following formula:

Soak 1 cup of raw nuts or seeds in water overnight. Drain. Blend nuts in a high-speed food processor with 3 to 4 cups of water ½ teaspoon pure vanilla, and sweetener to taste. Strain and serve.

You can make soy or almond milk at home. Following is a recipe for making soy milk from soy flour:

SOAK the soy flour in water for two hours to aid in smoothness and digestibility of the finished product. If in a hurry, boil the mix and soak it for a half-hour. Using one cup soy flour to three cups water, sprinkle the soy flour into boiling water, then SIMMER for 20 minutes, stirring occasionally. Strain through a fine sieve or cheesecloth.

You may prefer to sweeten the soymilk lightly, and/or add a pinch of salt, vanilla or other flavoring. For longest shelf life, COOL the mixture quickly such as by putting the hot milk container in a bowl of cold water, then refrigerate. It will stay fresh for at least four days, and even if it begins to sour it can be used in baking or to make soy yogurt.

If you have more time you can make soymilk from beans. To make about 3 quarts of soy milk, you will need:

- 1 cup of soybeans, organic if possible
- 11 total cups of water (to be added two to three cups at a time)
- Up to 1/4 cup of sweetener (according to your tastes)

Soak the beans in 2 cups of water overnight for a minimum of 10 hours. They should be doubled, or more, in size after soaking. The container should be large enough to allow the beans to expand. Use cheesecloth or muslin cloth for straining. To reduce the "beanie" taste you can remove the outer skins after soaking if you wish to take the time.

Pour the water the soybeans were soaking in plus the soybeans into the blender. Add four cups of water and blend until smooth.

Pour the soybean mixture into cheesecloth and hold over the pot. Squeeze out as much liquid as you can. After, pour the leftover soybean pulp back into the blender and add 3 more cups of water and blend until smooth. Repeat straining the mixture through the cheesecloth. Pour the pulp into the blender again and add 2 more cups of water (this brings you to 11 total cups). Strain the mixture again.

Put the pot on the stove top and turn the heat to high. Stir the mixture until it comes to a boil. Be sure to keep the soy milk from sticking to the bottom of the pot. Skim foam off the top. Boil the mixture for 2-3 minutes.

Add about 1/4 cup of sweetener to taste (1 teaspoon per cup). Other flavors can also be used to flavor soy milk such as vanilla, chocolate or fruits).

Soy milk can be enjoyed either hot or cold. Thickness can be adjusted by adding or reducing water. It can be stored in the refrigerator for up to one week.

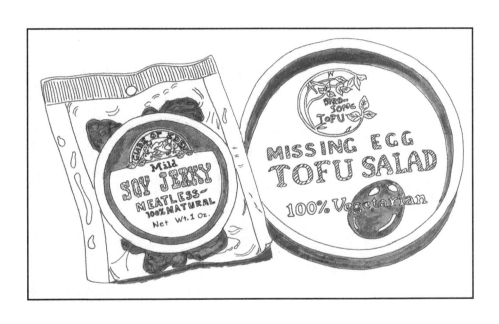

More Soy

The soybean is a noble and versatile bean. We eat soybeans in burritos or burgers or straight form the bowl. In our dairy we produce soymilk, which we drink and make into ice cream, yogurt, frogurt [frozen yogurt], tofu, tempeh [cultured soybean cake] and other soy cheeses. We also make soybeans into tempeh, a very tasty cultured bean cake.

--The Farm Vegetarian Cookbook

An increasing variety of soy products can be found in supermarkets and stores like Trader Joes, including, besides the familiar soy "veggie" burgers, soy cream cheese, soy corn dogs, soy lunch "meats," soy breakfast sausage and soy hot dogs. There are restaurants featuring soy creations on their menus that mimic all the familiar meat, fish and cheese entrees, but transformed into vegetarian offerings. Tofu, which is boiled, curdled, and pressed, similar to dairy cheese, can be made into many dishes including sweet ones like tofu cheesecake. There are also simple recipes using soy you can use at home.

SOYMILK PUDDING

To make a soymilk pudding from hot soymilk, simply put strained soymilk back into the pan and add 2 or 3 tablespoons of arrowroot powder which has first been mixed with cold water to form a smooth paste so that the mixture will not lump. Briefly boil the mixture until it begins to thicken (remember soymilk boils over easily if not carefully stirred and watched), then remove from heat. As the pudding cools you may add vanilla, honey or fructose, carob powder, fruit juice or any other flavorings your individual taste and imagination inspire.

A note about thickeners: the most commonly used thickener for hot liquids is cornstarch. However, processes involved in the production of cornstarch make it something some might wish to avoid. First, since the advent of genetically modified organisms, or GMOs, almost all cornstarch is now made from corn that has been genetically engineered. Many people concerned about their health seek to avoid GMOs in their diet, and many products sold by health-conscious companies exclude GMOs. You can buy non-GMO cornstarch but it is usually more expensive. The process of extracting cornstarch can be quite harsh as well, using chemicals and high heat to transform the corn into a powder. Arrowroot, derived from a South American tuber using natural processing, works just as well as a thickening agent and is generally the more healthful choice.

You can make an "instant" soy pudding from soy flour:

1 ½ T arrowroot
3 T honey
2 T soy flour
1 cup cold water
1 T oil (optional)

Mix ingredients thoroughly in a pan then heat slowly until thickened, stirring constantly.

SOY YOGURT

Soak soybeans for 24 hours, changing the water every 4 hours or so, then finally draining. Blend until creamy using equal parts water and soybeans. Add yogurt starter or mix in some commercial plain yogurt that does not contain gelatin. Or start with ready-made plain soymilk. You can then follow the incubation methods detailed for SEED YOGURT in the Fermented Foods chapter.

A few words about tofu can serve as a basic guide to this versatile protein dish. The first mention of tofu goes back to a Chinese text dating from 950 AD! Benjamin Franklin is the earliest known American to write about tofu, in a letter mailed from London to Philadelphia in 1770. Tofu is now sold widely in health food stores, supermarkets, and specialty stores like Whole Foods and Trader Joes. Most common is the water-packed soft tofu, which can also be found in organic versions. It is also sold in "medium" and "firm' variations.

Before cooking with tofu the blocks should be drained by placing them on an absorbent surface such as layered paper towels or a dish towel for 5-10 minutes. You can also freeze a whole block of tofu, though with this method it's best to cut the block into the sizes you want beforehand. It's best to drain the tofu first, to avoid ending up with an icy block. Freezing pulls out almost all the moisture, compacting the curds and extracting the whey, leaving behind a spongy product that readily absorbs sauces. Frozen tofu can be defrosted in the fridge, microwave, or tossed into boiling water. Here are descriptions of the degrees of firmness:

Soft: Its similarity to soft desserts makes soft tofu a great neutral base for both sweet and savory dishes. Because it has a high water content, soft tofu is not recommended for shallow frying—the sputtering and spit-back can be dangerous.

Medium: A good choice for dishes that don't require much manipulation, as when braising or boiling. Because there is more whey in medium-firm tofu, it may break up during vigorous stir-frying.

Firm: Holds up quite well to frying and stuffing. It can be battered, crusted, baked, boiled, pan-fried, stir-fried, deep-fried, or glazed .

Silken: Because curds never form, this style of tofu—be it soft, firm or extra firm—has a smooth and "silky" appearance. More delicate than a block tofu, silken tofu requires delicate handling, lest it fall apart. It is particularly suited to saucy recipes such as dressings, smoothies, and egg or yogurt substitutions.

There are even more varieties of tofu to discover and enjoy, including fresh silken/custard tofu, dry five spice tofu that comes in the form of a bean cake, smoked tofu which is smoked in tea leaves and very firm, and salty prepared fried tofu pockets, called *inari*. This Japanese snack is made of deep fried tofu that's been puffed up and hollowed out, like pita bread, then simmered in a sugar and soy sauce.

With all these delicious varieties of soy, who needs meat or dairy products?

Food Logic and Consumerism

The earlier chapter "Food Horror Stories," highlighted foods that sensible people would want to avoid. We can turn to what foods can be sought out for better health. Some will be familiar to many, others less so. Besides examining labels on products to discover any ingredients you would prefer to avoid, which is a good habit to acquire, the consumer should realize that not all versions of food are the same nutritionally.

A prime example concerns bread. There is a reason why health-conscious people choose whole wheat bread, because the standard "enriched flour" loaves are nearly nutritionally worthless. To produce "enriched" flour, processors take the natural wheat berry and strip off the hard outer coating of bran (which they may use as an ingredient for high-fiber versions of foods). They remove the wheat germ, which contains beneficial wheat germ oil but presents the disadvantage of rapid spoilage; they may sell that wheat germ separately as a toasted product. So now they get extended *shelf life*—a very important consideration in the commercial food business, which refers to the amount of time a product can sit on the shelf waiting to be purchased before it spoils. Then they work with what is left: the starchy inner berry or endosperm.

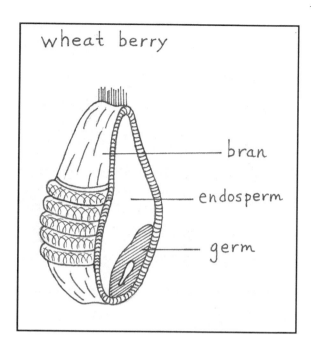

In contrast, when making whole wheat bread, the entire wheat berry with all of its nutrients is used. By fracturing the berry and using only the starchy part, the following will get lost nutritionally:

- Half of the beneficial unsaturated fatty acids
- Virtually all of the vitamin E
- Fifty percent of the calcium
- Seventy percent of the phosphorus
- Eighty percent of the iron
- Ninety eight percent of the magnesium
- Fifty to 80 percent of the B vitamins

(Dr. Joseph Mercola, *The Little-Known Secrets about Bleached Flour.* Mercola.com March 26, 2009)

Then comes bleaching. The starchy flour is put through a chlorine gas bath to both whiten and "age" the product. 100 years ago, before this process was invented, all flour was unbleached and aged for several months to improve gluten and baking quality. Now, using chlorine gas as a bleaching and oxidizing agent quickly (within 48 hours) produces similar results. Other chemicals and chemical salts may also be used for this purpose. A byproduct of the bleaching process is *alloxan*, which may be linked to the onset of diabetes.

Note that bleached white flour production is not done to serve consumers, but to increase shelf life by retarding spoilage and to make the bread look white and "clean." In France the only ingredients for bread permitted by law are flour, water, yeast and salt—certainly not chemical additives. The chemical azodicarbonamide, for example, is banned in Europe and Australia but routinely used in the U. S. Another problem derives from the fact that white bread is made using only the starch. Since the endosperm functions as a carbohydrate food supply for the growing wheat seed, those carbs when eaten rapidly break down into units of sugar, leading to dangerous spikes and crashes in blood sugar levels.

A further consideration is that today's flour mills are designed for mass-production, using high-temperature, high-speed steel rollers, so in the process of making flour heat sensitive nutrients are destroyed. A better method that preserves more nutrients is stone milling, which was for millennia the only way to grind flour. When roller milling was adopted about a century ago, some people protested on health grounds, including Dr. Harvey Wiley, first head of the FDA. But clearly when it comes to most commercial bread, efficiency won out over nutrition. Sprouted grain bread is another improvement over conventional milled flour. Soaking grains in water until they begin to sprout releases enzymes that break down protein and carbohydrates, making them easier to digest compared to milled grain, thus making available more nutrients. Widely available products known as Ezekiel or Genesis bread are made from sprouted grains and usually do not contain milled flour or preservatives. More information about sprouting and its benefits appears in the Sprouting chapter of this book.

When it comes to marketing food, it seems there is an inverse ratio between nutrition and the frequency of advertising. We don't expect to see ads on TV urging us to buy carrots, apples or bananas. But there are lots of ads for sugary breakfast cereals, fast food and salty snacks. While some popular alternative foods are gaining an ad profile such as some soy milk brands, the smaller food producers will be unable to hawk their products on the scale of General Mills. So don't expect to see ads for sprouted whole grain bread on prime time. Unfortunately one effect of such ad imbalance is that for many people the heavily advertised products become "normal" and acceptable, though if people understood what they were actually getting they might well seek out the lesser-known alternatives. In a certain way this principle holds true in the supermarket. Companies pay to put their products at eye-level, a practice known in the trade as 'slotting,' which are typically the big brands. Consumer advocates urge you to look up at the top shelves or down at the bottom to find the typically healthier, less-advertised alternatives, which often cost less too.

The power of advertising should not be underestimated. After all, in the last 30 years many of us have been persuaded to buy water in plastic bottles at a cost that is usually more than for gasoline, even though perfectly safe water flows from our taps at a fraction of the cost. If you are looking for change in the food industry, one very effective way is to vote with your consumer dollars. Over the 30 years since the first publication of *Oakland Organic*, the previous version of this book, the availability of alternative foods has expanded greatly, because a growing number of consumers desired soy milk or veggie burgers as just two examples. Rather than lose business to health food stores, supermarkets began carrying what people wanted to buy. The supermarket managers and buyers might have little interest in better nutrition, but you can count on them to have intense interest in their bottom line.

Advertisers employ sociologists, psychologists and marketing experts in their mission to persuade, and advertising can be fairly described as propaganda since it tries to manipulate consumers by any means short of some tactic that will bring trouble from the Federal Trade Commission. One campaign used this logic: "Kool-Aid; you loved it as a kid, you trust it as a mother." What is there to 'trust' about Kool-Aid, a product which boils down to powdered animal bones and artificial flavor and color to which the consumer adds sugar-water? What nutritional value could it have? What responsible mother would give such a product to her children rather than real fruit juice?

Even moms or dads looking for real fruit juice may be deceived. Many 'fruit drinks' on the supermarket shelf contain only between five to 15 percent fruit juice, may be sweetened with unhealthy additives such as high fructose corn syrup, and often contain artificial colors and preservatives. Kids may come to prefer these unnaturally sweet Frankenjuices to the real thing. Some health professionals worry that even 100% fruit juice can become a sugary habit if kids drink doses of it all day instead of water. Most bottled juices have been heated and pasteurized, a process which depletes most of the natural enzymes, vitamins and minerals. So in the end it's not terribly different from drinking sugar water, nutritionally speaking. To get the full value from juices you need to purchase a good juicer so that you can drink fresh fruit and vegetable juice as soon as possible after the whole fruits and vegetables have been processed. Freshly made juices, packed with live enzymes, vitamins and minerals, are alkalizing, provide intense hydration, and oxygenate cells and the bloodstream. A good juicing machine may cost in the neighborhood of $200, and they take some time to use, but clearly the health benefits are worth it. Lots of people go to commercial juice bars to get fresh juices, and those purchases add up over time. Also, some outlets use premixed "dairy base," artificial sweeteners or other ingredients you might avoid at home.

Consumers have been sold on convenience in general over nutritional considerations. Let's say you want to serve broccoli, but feel you don't have time to prepare the fresh vegetable. Instead you rummage in the freezer for the 'convenient' frozen package. This vegetable has already been chopped up (thoroughly oxidized, releasing forever delicate enzymes and vitamins), then cooked in a large vat of water, then drained (throwing away most of the nutrients which in overcooking have leached into the water), perhaps treated with questionable sauces or spices since the broccoli has now been rendered almost flavorless (salt, MSG, Hollandaise), then frozen.

When you take the 'vegetable' from your freezer, the directions tell you to recook it in too much water, drain it once more (lest any trace nutrients are still left in it) then serve it to yourself and your loved ones. And you still have the cooking pot to clean. Even microwaving means it has still been cooked twice over. The obvious question is whether this dish is worth serving at all, and it's little wonder your kids might not like their vegetables. And how much trouble is it to steam fresh broccoli? Put a half-inch of water into a pot, set the broccoli pieces on an inexpensive steamer device, and give it 8 or 10 minutes. You can do other things while the broccoli is steaming—you need not stand there and watch it. Steaming preserves the most nutritional value while cooking, does not generate much cleanup, and gives an appealing texture and flavor, as opposed to the overcooked, tasteless and over-salted or over-sauced frozen versions.

We could well question the whole idea that people are "saving time" by using frozen and other prepared foods, or by cruising the window of some fast food outlet. Even if preparing fresh foods takes more time, which it may or may not, the average American watches five hours of TV per day. And that's not counting time on the cell phone, going online, gaming, email and many other common daily screen activities. So why are people skimping on food preparation, settling for unhealthy quick foods and rushing through mealtimes? So they can get to their easy chairs in front of the TV faster? Shouldn't food be delicious, nutritious, and prepared so that it is worth enjoying? Shouldn't mealtimes include socializing, or even if eating alone, slowing down from daily routines and relaxing enough so that you can properly digest your food? And what is so undesirable about spending time in the kitchen? While cooking may not be everyone's cup of tea, we honor it as a creative art, celebrate celebrity chefs, and recognize 'foodies' whose passion is to enjoy and celebrate carefully prepared food.

It is doubtful consumers save money by buying fast and prepared foods. The concept behind selling commercially prepared foods is "value-added." So for example a company will buy dried corn, add salt and oil and flavorings, package it in microwaveable pouches, and sell it as popcorn for many times the price of the bulk corn. Or they will buy potatoes, one of the cheapest vegetables, process them, then sell them as instant mashed potatoes, French fries, or other varieties of convenience products, again for much more than the cost of the raw materials. So in the end we have all literally bought into a marketing scheme which is more about profits than either the well-being of or savings for consumers. Learning to appreciate fresher, more simply prepared foods means taking a significant step toward better health.

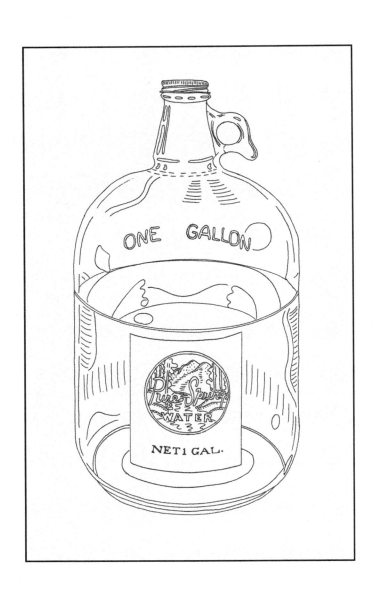

Fasting

"Fasting is the oldest therapeutic method known to man
[who] instinctively stopped eating when feeling ill and
abstained from food until his health was restored. Or perhaps
he learned this...from animals, which always fast when not
feeling well...nature...suggests to him to abstain from
eating by taking away his appetite for food...fasting has
such a profound rejuvenating effect of the functions of all
the vital organs, including the endocrine glands, which are
so decidedly responsible for how young or how old you feel
and look."

--Paavo Airola, Ph.D., N.D., *Are You Confused?* Phoenix:
Health Plus, 1987

Fasting has been used for religious and spiritual purification for centuries.
Christianity, Judaism, Gnosticism, Islam, Buddhism, Hinduism,
and American Indian traditions--all embrace fasting whether for
purification, spiritual vision, penance, mourning or sacrifice. Ghandi fasted
on different occasions up to 21 days at a time to win political concessions. The
farmworkers' leader Cesar Chavez undertook spiritual fasts including one of
25 days' duration in 1968 to promote the principle of nonviolence.

When you reflect on it for a moment, our bodies are designed to fast,
since in fact we do it every night while sleeping. In contemporary medicine,
fasting is required to get accurate readings for certain medical tests. Patients
are asked to do short fasts before tests for cholesterol and for blood sugar
levels, for example, to achieve a more accurate baseline count. People getting a
colonoscopy also are required to fast beforehand. The physician Joel Furman,

author of *Eat to Live: The Amazing Nutrient-Rich Program for Fast and Sustained Weight Loss and Fasting and Eating for Health,* writes that

> Americans eat 51% of their diet from processed foods and foods low in phytochemicals and antioxidants. So you see a buildup of waste products in the cells -- AGE, advanced glycation end products -- that build up in cellular tissues and lead to atherosclerosis, aging, diabetes, nerve damage, and the deterioration of organs. This is basic science and physiology every doctor learns in medical school.
>
> *(http://www.webmd.com/diet/is_fasting_healthy?page=2)*

Fasting, along with improving your overall diet, helps the body to remove that buildup of AGE waste products, according to Fuhrman and other fasting advocates.

How does fasting remove toxins from the body? When you go without eating for more than a day or two, the body enters into ketosis. Ketosis means when the body runs out of carbohydrates to burn for energy, it burns fat. "And the fat is where the body stores many of the toxins it absorbs from the environment," Fuhrman says. Fuhrman tells WebMD, he has seen fasting -- combined with improving the diet before and afterward -- eliminate lupus, arthritis and chronic skin conditions like psoriasis and eczema. He reports that fasting can heal the digestive tracts of those with ulcerative colitis and Crohn's disease, and lower blood pressure.

A fundamental lesson that fasting even for one day teaches us is that skipping a meal will not make most people faint or keel over (perhaps with the exception of those suffering from hypoglycemia). We need not necessarily "eat on the clock." There is no particular reason to break the fast which your body began when you went to sleep the night before as soon as you awake. There is no definitive scientific or medical evidence that eating breakfast is especially beneficial, or that it promotes healthy weight. Most likely the "breakfast at 8, lunch at noon, dinner at 6" pattern got ingrained in American culture as a result of the industrial revolution, when most workers wound up in a factory or on an office schedule. They eat before they leave home, eat lunch on their midday break, and eat dinner soon after they get home. But what might be healthier would be to eat when you are hungry, and not before.

Traditional eating patterns in other cultures and countries don't follow the American regimen. In Spain breakfast is typically a cup of coffee—perhaps accompanied by a churro. Lunch is the largest meal of the day, consisting of several courses, and eaten between 2 and 4 pm. Dinner is smaller-- a salad, a sandwich, or tapas, taken between 9 and 11 pm. The size pattern is similar in France, where breakfast is coffee and perhaps fruit or a croissant, and dinner is fruit or yogurt. So there is no set "healthy" pattern for times of day to eat, and if French or Spanish people just have coffee for breakfast and don't eat anything else until 2 pm, aren't they virtually fasting?

Fasting gives the body a rest from digestive processes; the body can then use that spare energy to cleanse itself on a cellular level. Waste products will be recirculated into the bloodstream to be eliminated through the skin, bladder, bowels and other organs of elimination during and immediately after the fast is broken.

There are variations for fasting, besides just the length of time it is done:

Fruit fasting (semi-fast): Eating dry fruit, fresh acidic fruit such as citrus and berries, or just melon as an aid to elimination.

Juice regimen: This might be an ideal fast for busy people or city dwellers, since it gives people some energy to go on. Citrus juices in particular, best diluted to half-strength with water, aid the body's eliminative system. You might also include vegetable broth, either homemade or using good vegetable cubes or powder (this book contains a chapter on broth). Some fasting experts recommend a mixture of fresh citrus juices and water with added sweetener for energy (honey, maple syrup or fructose), and perhaps a little cayenne pepper, and sipping this mixture throughout the day. The cayenne stimulates the circulatory system, aids digestion, helps regulate blood sugar, warms the body and kick-starts metabolism.

Water fast: Ingesting water only; distilled water is often recommended during a fast for its increased ability to bind to toxins, but not as a regular choice since it lacks minerals, can lead to loss of electrolytes, and may not have sufficient alkalinity. You might include herbal tea on a water fast unless you are trying to be a purist.

Dry fasting: This is clearly fasting at its most extreme, though it is sometimes undertaken for spiritual purposes. It is usually done for one day or less. One should be healthy and able to rest if attempting this complete denial of food and fluids to the body.

I have personally fasted short-term, for just a couple of days, on many occasions. Once I fasted for 20 days when I did not have to go to work or attend to any pressing business or commitments and could even visit the beach every day. I experienced no ill effects but rather a beneficial feeling. I "eased into" this long fast by simplifying my diet to salads and fruit for several meals before stopping solid food altogether. Then I began with juice fasting. After about a week of juice and broth I switched to water fasting for a few days, then did a dry fast for 24 hours, then went back to water, then juice, then finally after 20 days light eating of fruit and salads. I camped out under the stars during the time of the dry fast and felt a heightening of the senses along with spiritual connection to nature. Of course these are subjective impressions.

Following is a typical fasting routine. Be sure to scale down your eating to lighter, more easily digestible foods before undertaking the fast. The body takes varying time and effort to digest any substance, depending on its complexity and the number of processes necessary to break it down into usable form. Complex protein (meat, fish, even soy products) generally takes at least four hours for primary digestion in the stomach, often more. Starches take at least two to three hours. Simple fruits and vegetables usually take only one hour, and very juicy foods such as melons even less time. Juices pass through the body in about twenty minutes when taking nothing else.

Morning

Dry-fast for as long as is comfortable since that is what you have been doing all night anyway and you may find that once you start to drink you will feel thirsty and crave even more to drink.

Break the dry fast with lemon juice in warm water and perhaps honey or a little orange juice to sweeten to taste. For the rest of the day thirst can be quenched with small amounts of fruit juice, preferably fresh, diluted with three parts of water. Sparkling water may be especially satisfying and help to keep appetite in check.

Afternoon

At the end of the day or when returning from work, BROTH can be restorative and supply minerals as well as providing a savory drink at the time of day when one usually eats an evening meal. The broth can thickened and eaten slowly by spoonfuls to make it even more satisfying.

An 'on-the-go' substitute for broth could be low-sodium tomato or V-8 juice, though no canned product can compare nutritionally to fresh juices or to homemade broth.

Evening

If thirsty later in the evening, freshly juiced carrot and celery juice is satisfying. Other options for use during a liquid fast include:

> --herbal teas, perhaps sweetened with fructose or honey
> --sodas from health stores made without artificial ingredients or flavorings; ginger ale may work well, and there are ginseng sodas which may provide an energy boost
> --soy or rice milk if you feel you cannot stick to fasting without a drink that is more filling or satisfying than fruit juice and water.

The first day of fasting is often the hardest in terms of willpower and feelings of hunger. It may help to go out to a movie on the first evening of your fast to provide distraction, and to remove yourself from the vicinity of your refrigerator! Come home, go straight to bed, and when you wake up the next day you should find your appetite, even for liquids, will be greatly diminished. The fasting should become progressively easier with each additional day until self-control is no longer difficult. Your stomach may actually shrink when you stop eating solid food (there is both evidence for and medical debate about that), and eating less can help to reset your "appetite thermostat" so you won't feel as hungry and it will be easier to stick with fasting. Often the decision to see the fast through, and the control you ultimately have over when you stop, is enough to see it through to success.

Another helpful suggestion is to buy some psyllium seed powder (*plantago ovata*) or its equivalent. The powder can be mixed with juice or water and serves two main functions:

1) The moistened powder expands in your digestive tract to give a feeling of "bulk" and fullness which depresses the appetite.
2) The natural ingredients serve as a "digestive broom" to help the body loosen and eliminate wastes from the digestive tract.

Products of this type yield no ill effects and make initial fasting easier to see through. Psychologically, the investment in the product and commitment to the regimen which must be adhered to when using it are further aids to willpower.

How often should one fast? That depends on your goals. But a once a month, or even a once a week juice fast helps your organs rest from the chores of digestion and do some health-promoting detoxification. Fasting for three or four days will result in significantly more detoxification of the system, and some health authors recommend such a fast at the change of seasons. Even spending a day just eating fresh fruits and raw vegetables will give your body a period of rest and cleansing. While some people fast to achieve weight loss, as with all diets, if you go back to the same eating pattern you had before fasting, you will soon go back to the same weight you were before fasting, too.

Should you use an enema? If you are regularly eliminating during the fast, there is no need. Otherwise an enema will help, and inexpensive kits with easy instructions can be found at any drug store. If you are fasting for an extended period an enema every other day or so will aid the body in elimination.

Fasting can have short-term side effects such as headaches, dizziness, feeling lightheaded or fatigued, abnormal heart rhythms, low blood pressure, and a fruity taste in the mouth. You may also feel more sensitive to cold while fasting. If you plan a long fast, try to arrange it for a vacation time, preferably in warm weather and at a place with clean air and a restful atmosphere and environment. Rest as you feel you need to. Enjoy the exhilaration and self-respect you will feel!

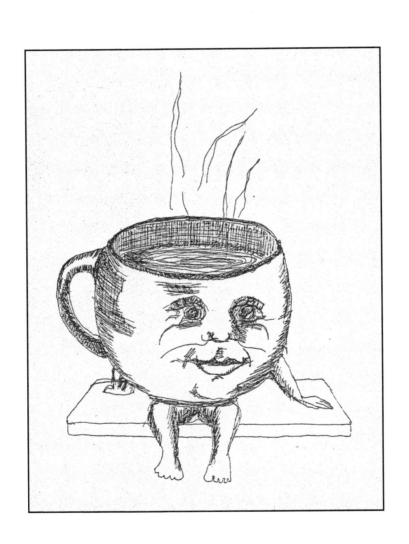

Broth

If you are fasting, or you don't feel as hungry as usual, or just want to eat more lightly than having a full meal, you can make a mineral-rich and satisfying broth. A separate chapter of this book takes up the topic of minerals, which are a vital and often overlooked aspect of good nutrition, and making broth is a delicious opportunity to ensure that you are getting enough. Of course you can purchase bouillon cubes, miso soup powders and other "instant" versions of broth, but this can be a much more flexible and healthful recipe. In cold weather broth can be made thicker and more substantial; in warm weather it can be made lighter, like a fine consommé.

What follows is a recipe outline for making broth, but you will discover your own variations.

> Start with vegetable bouillon cubes or get a jar of vegetable base or paste. Remember many commercial bouillon cubes use beef or chicken as ingredients and they can be overly salted or contain other undesirable ingredients. Look for vegetarian cubes or jars; you may find these in supermarket soup sections, or you may need to shop at a health store. Many health stores also sell 'vegetable protein broth powder' in bulk, preferably without added salt, so you can sample different offerings and select one that suits your personal tastes. These powders are made from dried or dehydrated vegetables, which even without added salt provide enough sodium and lend lots of flavor too.

The powder, cubes and/or paste can be dissolved in hot water to form the basic broth. For even more nutrition, you can use *rejuvelac* (see Sprouting chapter), or the cooking liquid left over from steaming vegetables. Some people cook a variety of vegetables in a pot and then save the liquid to use as soup base.

To this basic broth you can add any or all of the following:

Kelp (seaweed) powder or flakes or even whole pieces of seaweed if desired; you can find seaweed in a variety of shapes and colors

Miso (fermented rice of bean paste), best first melted in warm water and added <u>after</u> the broth is cooked

Soy sauce or its variations, including Bragg Liquid Aminos that contains 16 amino acids

Tomato juice (fresh if possible), or tomato paste for body and flavor

Spices and seasonings such as basil leaves, parsley flakes, dill, oregano, or dried seasoning mixes; rubbing between your palms to crush leaves will release more flavor

Yeast powder or flakes which are full of B vitamins (see separate chapter in this book); this can be added in the same manner as for miso, dissolving in warm water then stirring in after the broth is cooked

Peanut or almond butter which add protein and flavor and act as a thickening agent; can be added the same way as for miso and yeast.

This recipe can be made into a thickened soup by using more tomato paste and/or thickening with a tablespoon or more (depending on how much broth you are preparing) of cornstarch or arrowroot powder dissolved first in a little cold water, then stirred in and simmered for a few minutes until thickened. Again, if you are adding miso, yeast or nut butter those are best added after this process, waiting for a few minutes after bringing the broth to a boil to thicken to let it cool some before stirring in these last few ingredients.

This recipe can be made quickly, but if you have more time, try making broth from fresh vegetables. The nutrition guru Paavo Airola promoted what he called Potassium Broth as an **alkalizing drink** and an **electrolyte balancer** that helps cells function optimally, and can be particularly soothing at the end of a stressful day. Potassium gives a special energy boost to the brain, as well as to the beat of the heart.

Here is his Soup of Life recipe:

- 2-3 quarts of water
- A few potatoes
- A couple of celery stalks
- a couple carrots

   To that, add leafy vegetables such as collard, chard, kale, sunflower greens, broccoli, zucchini, beet tops or cabbage. Bring to a boil and then cover and simmer slowly for a half hour, then let stand for another half hour. Any unused portion can be refrigerated then warmed later to serve.

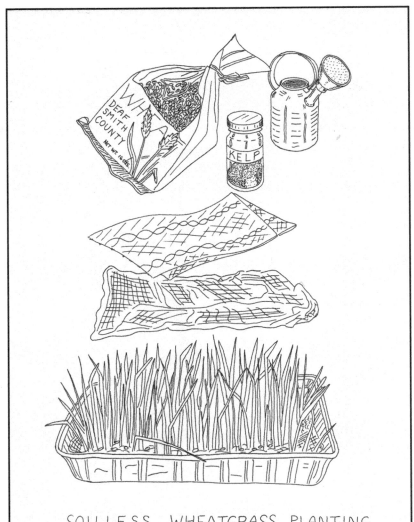

SOILLESS WHEATGRASS PLANTING

Wheatgrass and Chlorophyll

"City dwellers are exposed to radiation from strontium 90, iodine 131, fluorescent lights, x-rays and radioactive pollutants. The solid content of wheatgrass juice is up to 70% chlorophyll...Chlorophyll can regenerate the bloodstream... Other studies have shown chlorophyll in live food to greatly increase survival of those exposed to lethal radiation."

--Victoras Kulvinskas, *Love Your Body,*
21st Century Bookstore, 1972

What is wheatgrass? It is grass grown by sprouting wheat (rye, barley, alfalfa, oats and other grains may also be used). Wheatgrass juice contains chlorophyll, the chemical in plants that makes them green and also allows them to make energy from sunlight through photosynthesis. Chlorophyll is an effective blood cleanser, with a molecular structure nearly identical to that of hemoglobin. Since the first publication of this book the benefits of wheatgrass have become much more widely known, so that many people can buy it over the counter in commercial juice bars. In addition, stores like Trader Joes, other health-oriented stores, and now even supermarkets sell "green juices" made with chlorophyll-rich ingredients such as spirulina, chlorella and barley grass.

Dr. Chiu-Nan of the University of Texas System Cancer Center reported that "extracts of wheat sprouts exhibit antagonistic activity toward known carcinogens." (Chiu-Nan Lai et al: *The inhibitions of in vitro metabolic activation of carcinogens by wheat sprout extracts.* Nutrition & Cancer, 1978,1(1) Fall: 27 – 30). According to WedMD, wheatgrass can be beneficial for a long list of conditions, including

--removing deposits of drugs, heavy metals, and cancer-causing agents from the body

--removing toxins from the liver and blood

--preventing gray hair, reducing high blood pressure, improving digestion, and lowering cholesterol by blocking its absorption

--treating various disorders of the urinary tract, and treating respiratory tract complaints including coughs and the common cold

--alleviating joint pain and chronic skin problems

--and treating cancer and arthritis in alternative treatment programs

(http://www.webmd.com/vitamins-supplements/ ingredientmono-1073-wheatgrass)

People, and particularly city dwellers, are typically exposed on a daily basis to radon, x-rays, cigarette smoke, UV rays, cosmic radiation due to elevation, radiation and other pollutants from both coal and nuclear power plants within 50 miles, air pollution and air particulates. There are still at least 1700 Superfund sites in the U. S., the worst toxic waste sites, most located near large population centers. About 11 million people in the U.S., including 3 to 4 million children, live within 1 mile of a federal Superfund site. Our Environmental Protection Agency lists as common contaminants from Superfund sites asbestos, lead, dioxin, mercury, and radiation.

In light of this information, it makes good sense to include foods like wheatgrass and miso (detailed in the Fermented Foods chapter) which can strip heavy metals and cancer-causing agents from the body. They will also give you renewed energy, and they can serve as a kind of nutritional insurance policy if you are not getting your fair share of fresh greens.

It is simple and inexpensive to grow wheatgrass in your own kitchen:

Buy wheat berries (the part of the wheat ground to make bread flours) from any health store or supermarket selling bulk foods. They are quite inexpensive in bulk, and can be purchased in large quantities since these seeds keep for years. Arrowhead Mills and Bobs Red Mill are sample brands which can be found in many stores. Remember, other grains such as rye or barley can also be used.

Soak the wheat berries in tepid water overnight (about 12 hours), or for 24 hours in winter. You can save the soak water to use on houseplants, for soup stock, or you can ferment it to make rejuvilac (see Fermented Foods chapter) by letting it stand in a warm place for another 36 hours. The soak water is full of vitamins and minerals.

Using aluminum foil baking trays (from any supermarket),

1) line them with paper towels to insure that seeds get water
2) add a layer of cheesecloth (available at supermarkets and even auto stores)
3) spread soaked seeds in a dense layer one-seed deep in the prepared trays
4) irrigate with some of the soak water
5) sprinkle with dulse (dried seaweed powder) which acts as a fertilizer to aid growth
6) slip the prepared tray(s) into plastic produce bags and put in a warm place away from direct sunlight for two or three days

Usually the trays will need no further watering, but check to make sure the seeds stay moist. After green sprouts and small blades appear, take the trays out of the plastic bags and put in sunlight until grass reaches 6 to 8 inches in height. Keep moist; spraying with a plant mister will also improve your crop.

The least expensive way to harvest and consume your fresh wheatgrass is to use a blender. While this is not ideal, since blending aerates, dilutes and slightly heats the juice, depleting some of the nutrients, it is nevertheless practical for most kitchens. Simply cut grass close to roots with scissors and put in blender with enough water (or fresh carrot or celery juice) to allow the blender blades to crush the grass. Strain out pulp and enjoy.

Even if you don't have a blender the plain blades of wheat grass can be chewed (spit out the pulp) or used on salads—teeth are an effective, free juicer. As a bonus, wheatgrass juice can help prevent tooth decay!

If you are planning to grow your own wheatgrass regularly you will want to purchase a grass juicer. The two basic types to consider are a manual juicer, which resembles a miniature meat grinder (though obviously that's where the resemblance stops!) and start at about $50 for a good machine. These can only be used for juicing wheatgrass, but they hardly generate any heat and are easy to clean. The other choice is a masticating electric juicer, of which some models can also serve as a general juicer for fruits and vegetables. These will cost upwards of $200, though given that they can also be used for general juicing they can be a great investment in your health.

Other sources of concentrated chlorophyll are dried spirulina or barley grass, which are sold in both powder and capsule or tablet forms. Both are full of enzymes, amino acids, vitamins and minerals, and of course chlorophyll. Spirulina is a blue-green algae that grows on the surfaces of tropical and subtropical lakes and ponds. Records of the Spanish conquistadors indicate that spirulina was used as a food source for the Aztecs and other Mesoamericans until the 16th century. It was also traditionally harvested by the Kanembu people of Central Africa from small lakes and ponds around what is now called Lake Chad. Legend has it that the Aztecs carried dried spirulina into battle because it was easy to carry and so nourishing that they could live on it exclusively for days. Dried spirulina contains about 60% protein. It is a complete protein containing all essential amino acids. Spirulina intake has also been found to prevent damage caused by toxins affecting the heart, liver, kidneys, neurons, eyes, ovaries, DNA, and testicles.

Barley grass is also a great choice when it comes to concentrated chlorophyll. Barley grass is about 45% protein and contains, among other beneficial substances, 11 times the amount of calcium than there is in cow's milk, 5 times the iron content of spinach, and close to seven times the vitamin C in oranges, along with up to 1,000- beneficial enzymes which help in essential cell regulation.

Spirulina and barley grass can also be used for fasting since each provides many nutrients yet can easily be mixed with liquids. Those fasting may experience less discomfort from hunger and fatigue when taking these supplements during a fast.

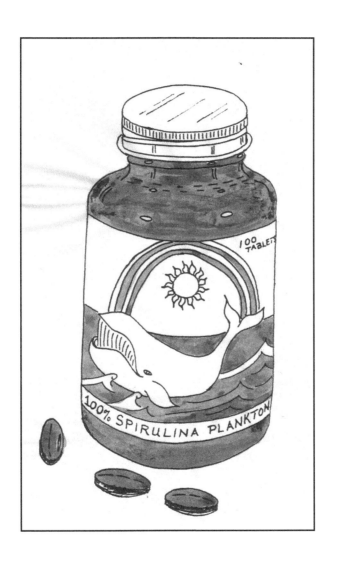

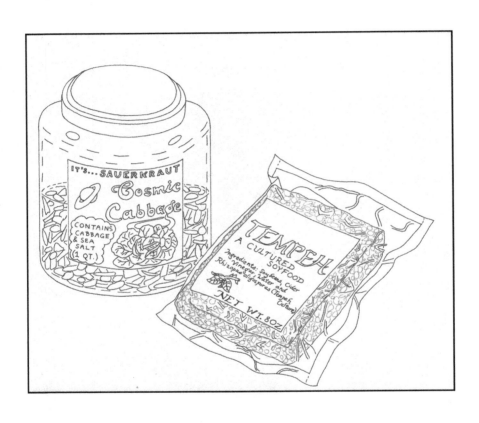

Fermented Foods

Fermented foods have been a staple of the human diet for millennia. They range from the commonplace to the more exotic. Most people have eaten sauerkraut or yogurt or perhaps buttermilk or bleu cheese crumbled on a salad or sourdough bread. Many cheeses are fermented, and even coffee beans and beer undergo a fermentation process. Fermentation is a process in which food is exposed to bacteria and yeasts, by inoculation or naturally through the air. Beneficial microorganisms prevail over harmful ones, consuming carbohydrates in the food. The results are interesting flavors, textures, and smells. Before the invention of refrigeration such a process was the only way to extend the life of perishables. And fermented foods that have not been cooked (which kills off the beneficial bacteria) are really good for you.

We harbor beneficial bacteria in our own gut to improve digestion and boost immunity. Fermented foods are loaded with probiotics, good bacteria which encourage the growth of the beneficial bacteria already in your system. For example, *lactobacillus bulgaris*, the bacteria found in yogurt culture, destroys putrefactive bacteria in the digestive tract and promotes growth of 'friendly' acidophilus bacteria that in turn help to manufacture B vitamins, and vitamin K which helps prevent arterial plaque buildup and heart disease. Such culture is also a natural antibiotic, killing virulent bacteria such as streptococcus, typhus and staphylococcus.

Buttermilk, kefir, yogurt and other traditional fermented foods made from dairy milk possess similar healthful properties, but the use of dairy products themselves poses health problems (see Dairy Products chapter). Yet you need not forgo the wonderful flavors and many benefits of cultured or fermented milk products. The same types of food can be easily made using soy milk, rice milk, almond milk, coconut milk and other mixes. Non-dairy yogurt, if labeled "live and active cultures," delivers 100 million probiotic cultures per gram. Other food and beverages, with samples listed below, have the same healthful properties and can easily be made a regular part of your diet.

Sauerkraut, made from just cabbage and salt, delivers probiotics and fiber.

Miso, fermented paste made from barley, rice or soybeans, high in sodium, adds lots of flavor to soups and other dishes.

Tempeh, which is like very firm tofu, is made from naturally fermented soybeans and has a slightly nutty flavor; it delivers complete protein with all essential amino acids and is a good source of probiotics.

Kombucha is a fermented tea drink which has been around for centuries but recently became popular in the U.S. and has beneficial bacteria similar to yogurt, kefir, or other probiotic drinks; most probiotic benefits come with *unpasteurized* kombucha, though that can raise some safety issues and there are commercially prepared pasteurized versions.

Miso is especially interesting. This food originated in China during the 3rd century BC and was probably introduced to Japan at the same time as Buddhism in the 6th century AD. In an extraordinary book by the Japanese doctor Tatsuichiro Akizuki entitled *Nagasaki 1945*, he gives an account of how the roof of his hospital was blown away by the blast of the atomic bomb (which had a plutonium core) dropped on that city at the end of WWII. In the days immediately following the bombing little help arrived from beyond the devastated city. The principle food Akizuki had on hand was a supply of brown rice balls and miso, which he continued feeding to his patients and staff as they remained on the hospital site, despite the radiation hazard which was little understood at the time. During the weeks and months following the bombing, hundreds if not thousands of people died of radiation effects, but none of Dr. Akizuki's patients, who were eating primarily the brown rice and miso soup, died of radiation poisoning.

> The radioactivity may not have been a fatal dose [Akizuki writes] but I, and other staff members and in-patients kept on living on the lethal ashes of the bombed ruins. It was thanks to this salt mineral method that all of us survived disaster free from severe symptoms of radiation.
>
> (*Nagasaki 1945*. London: Quartet Books, 1981)

The protective properties of miso were confirmed in 1972 when researchers discovered that it contains dipicolonic acid, an alkaloid that chelates heavy metals, such as radioactive strontium, and discharges them from the body. Subsequent research has shown that miso also protects against some forms of cancer and heart disease and cancels out the effects of some carcinogens.

While brown rice is not a fermented food, it is worth mentioning here that it too, as Dr. Akizuki found, indeed helps in the prevention of various cancers such as colon cancer, breast cancer and leukemia. Leukemia is particularly associated with radiation poisoning which was found to still affect some survivors of the WWII bombing as long as 50 years later. The beneficial properties of brown rice are attributed to potent antioxidants and high fiber content in the brown rice. The fiber content of brown rice has the ability to bind itself to harmful cancer- causing toxins in the body. This prevents the toxins from attaching to the walls of the colon and helps eliminate them from the body.

For those who wish to make homemade yogurt and other fermented foods, some recipes follow here.

SEED YOGURT

½ cup raw sunflower and/or sesame seeds
11/2 cups water
2 T commercial yogurt (made without vegetable gum) or yogurt starter (available in dried form)

Grind seeds in a blender, then add ½ cup water and starter and blend to a creamy consistency, gradually adding the rest of the water. Incubate in 1) a box with an electric bulb; 2) in sunlight or a warm part of the house; 3) submerged in warm water, perhaps in the oven with the pilot light on. Pouring the mixture into jars rinsed with boiling water and incubating for 5 to 9 hours should result in a thickened, delicious seed yogurt.

This mixture will ferment without any yogurt or starter—simply allow maximum time. Using rejuvelac (recipe appears below) in place of all or part of the water will cut fermentation time.

Almonds, cashews, pumpkin seeds, walnuts and other nuts can be used, preferably in combination with sweet-flavored sunflower seeds.

SEED CHEESE can be made using the above directions but reducing liquid to one cup.

RAW TOFU

1 cup soybeans   3 cups water

Rinse beans and soak for 12 hours. Rinse, then soak again for another 12 hours. Wash, then blend soaked beans with 2 cups of water or rejuvelac until creamy. Incubate 4 to 8 hours. Press through cheesecloth—save whey for sauces and soups. Nutritionally superior to cooked tofu!

REJUVELAC

1 cup wheat or other seed (hulled millet, oats, rice barley, rye)
2 cups water; spring water, filtered water or distilled are best

Wash the wheat or other seed then soak in a jar for two or three days at room temperature. You will notice fine effervescence or bubbles and can begin drinking the now-lemony fermented beverage which contains many nutrients. Don't let fermentation go on to the point where the rejuvelac sours—test it now and then. You can pour off the liquid and store and extra in the refrigerator. Replace water to previous level and you can reuse the seed for up to two weeks if it is of high quality. Eden Foods, Bob's Red Mill and Arrowhead are examples of quality grains that will work well.

QUICK SAUERKRAUT

If you want to speed up the fermentation, you can start by buying a jar of Bubbies or similar traditionally fermented sauerkraut and then use the juice from that. This recipe will fill a 5-gallon crock, or can be scaled down.

1. Sanitize crock and utensils in dishwasher or with boiling water.
2. Remove outer leaves and cores from cabbage.
3. Thinly slice cabbage--using a food processor greatly speeds this up!
4. As you slice, mix 4 T salt with every 5 lbs. of cabbage and let stand in a bowl to wilt a little
5. When juice starts to form on cabbage/salt mixture, pack tightly into crock using sanitized utensils or clean hands.
6. Repeat this until cabbage is within about 4-5 inches of top of container.
7. Pack down until water level rises above cabbage and all cabbage is entirely submerged
8. If there is not enough liquid to cover cabbage, make a brine with 1½ T salt in 1 quart of water. Add cooled brine to crock until all cabbage is completely covered.
9. Once cabbage is submerged, fill a 2-gallon food-grade freezer bag with 2 quarts of water. Place inside another 2 gallon bag.
10. Place brine-filled bag on top of cabbage in crock, making sure that it touches all edges and prevents air from reaching cabbage.
11. Cover crock with plastic wrap and cloth or towel. Tie tightly.

12. Put crock in an area that will stay between 70 and 75 degrees.
13. Fermentation will begin within a day and take 3-5 weeks depending on temperature.
14. After 3 weeks, check for desired tartness. If you are going to can, make it slightly more tart than usual as it will lose some tartness. Once fermented, it can be eaten right away, or frozen or canned.

This recipe comes from WellnessMama.com

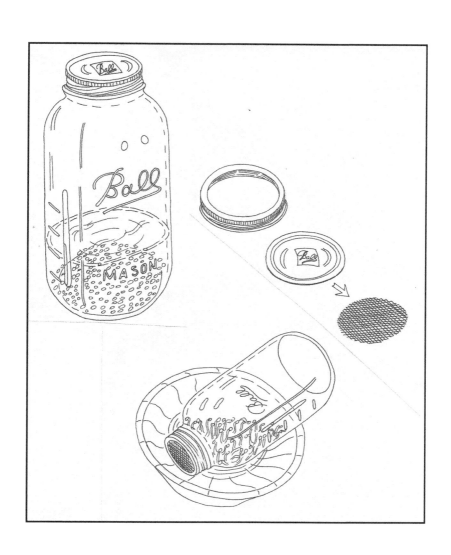

Sprouting

Sprouting is one of the simplest and most nutritionally rewarding procedures in vegetarian food preparation. By sprouting, one pound of dry seed is converted into six to eight pounds of living food, food which provides protein, vitamins, essential amino acids and chlorophyll, not to mention roughage. Sprouts require no energy to grow and can be consumed raw (you may prefer to cook heavier seed slightly, such as peas and lentils).

Sprouts also contain digestive enzymes and some of the highest known levels of certain antioxidants. One cup of sprouts provides 119 percent of your daily allotment of vitamin C. Certain compounds are *not* contained in sprouts which makes them healthier, such as tannins which are present in seeds but eliminated during the soaking step done prior to sprouting. Sprouting whole grains reduces the amount of starch they contain and boosts their nutritional value. An advantage to sprouted wheat, rye and barley is that they contain less of the protein gluten, which is difficult for some people to digest.

All you need are seeds of your choice:

alfalfa	sunflower seeds	soybeans
mung	whole dried peas	wheat
lentils	radish	raw peanuts

Any of these, or mixtures of these or others, plus a large glass jar and some cheesecloth or other screening and you are ready to sprout.

Wash the seeds, then soak overnight (5 to 8 hours) in spring or distilled water. Ordinary tap water may cause some seeds to not germinate; some blades of wheatgrass added to tap water will help. When you drain seeds the next day or after the soaking period, you can use the soak liquid in broth or other recipes or drink it as is—it contains many nutrients in its own right. Houseplants will also benefit from watering with this soak-liquid.

Screen the mouth of the jar using a layer of cheesecloth and a rubber band (or use a "ball" type canning jar with fine-mesh stainless steel cut to fit the ring) and invert the wet seeds so that excess water drains. Setting the jar at a tilt in a heavy bowl is fine, or even in your dish drainer, provided it is not in bright light. The seeds will sprout faster if they are started in low light but kept at room temperature.

Rinse the seeds morning and night--a simple procedure, as there is no need to remove the screen. Just pour water into the jar to wet the seeds, then invert again. In two or three days the seeds should have germinated and sprouted, becoming seedlings. At this point they will grow in light, and in 3 to 4 days, just before they are ready to eat, be sure to put them in the window or out in sunlight for a few hours to increase the chlorophyll value of the sprouts. They will turn much greener on the last day.

Sprouts can be stored in the refrigerator in plastic or in the covered container for several days. If you want to use them up in a hurry, put them in the blender with enough water to liquefy, then strain out the liquid and drink, or use them in broth, sauces or salad dressing.

Be sure to get the best (organic if possible) seeds available. They are an inexpensive commodity, often sold in bulk in food stores, and can even be purchased by the pound in feed stores to get them more cheaply. Just be sure that none of the seeds have been treated with mercury, a deadly poison.

Wheat berries, the dry seeds from which flour is ground, can also be sprouted and put to multiple uses. Rye, triticale and other related grains (such as barley or millet) can be used the same way:

> Proceed as for seed sprouting, and "harvest" as soon as the berries begin to germinate—little white sprouts will appear, and should be no longer than the seed itself.

Sprouted berries can be used for making **sunbread:**

> Put sprouted berries in blender or a grain mill and crush, using enough water to moisten well. Spread this mixture (seasoned with kelp, soy sauce, paprika or other herbs OR

mixed with soaked raisins or currants or dates to make a sweet version) on oiled foil pans in one of two ways:

1) Thinly, about ½ inch deep, for sun-drying—simply set in sunlight until dry on top, turn with spatula (break up or cut into pieces if necessary to turn) and dry the other side. Use a very low oven if no sunlight is available.

2) Thickly, in a baking tray or dish; put in 325 degree oven for about one hour, until dry on crust but moist inside. This is "Wayfarers" type bread, but made much more inexpensively than similar commercial versions sold in stores.

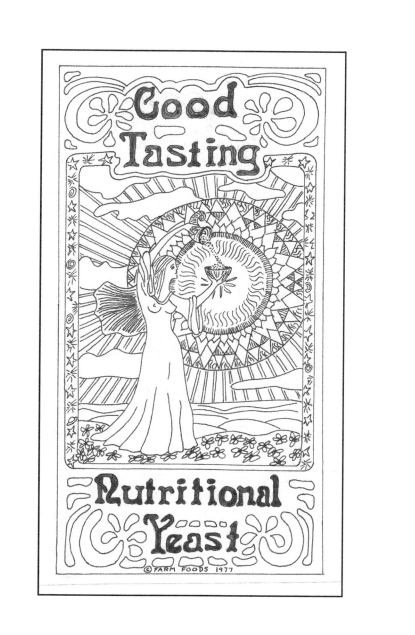

Good Tasting

Nutritional Yeast

© FARM FOODS 1977

Yeast

Most people think of yeast as something to make home-made bread rise. Nutritional yeast, meant to be eaten as a food, differs from brewer's yeast used in baking. It is sold in the form of flakes or as a yellow powder and can be found in the bulk section of most natural food stores. Nutritional yeast has a flavor that is described as nutty, cheesy, or creamy, which makes it popular as an ingredient in cheese substitutes. It is often used by vegans in place of cheese. It can be used in many recipes such as in mashed and fried potatoes, in soups and gravies, and atop scrambled tofu. Another popular use is as a topping for popcorn. Nutritional yeast is produced by culturing in a nutrient medium for several days. The primary ingredient in the growth medium is glucose, usually from either sugarcane or beet molasses. When the yeast is ready, it is deactivated with heat and then harvested, washed, dried and packaged. Nutritional yeast is an excellent source of iron, magnesium, phosphorus, zinc, chromium, selenium, and other minerals as well as 18 amino acids, protein, folic acid, biotin, and other vitamins.

Nutritional yeast is a good source of B vitamins, and in particular B-12, which is particularly important for vegans. Vitamin B12 is crucial to the human body, necessary to produce new DNA, red blood cells, proteins, hormones and lipids (fats). Vitamin B12 is also key to the health of nerves. While trace amounts of B-12 are available in many common foods, the hygienic nature of American packaging and food processing can deprive consumers of B-12. For example, in countries with less fastidious practices B-12 is provided by residual insect remains on food. Unbeknownst to many consumers, The U. S. Department of Agriculture officially allows "acceptable levels of filth" in foods, now referred to as Food Defect Action Levels. Foods as ordinary as chocolate, peanut butter and flour contain a tiny percentage of insect parts that are considered harmless and actually add some nutrition to the food.

In general, vitamin B12 is found in animal products, so it is a good idea for strict vegetarians and vegans to supplement their intake of B-12. Nutritional yeast is the best vegetarian source of vitamin B12. Just 2 teaspoons (6 grams) a day of nutritional yeast should cover an adult's vitamin B12 needs. Additionally, most multivitamins contain the daily recommended amount of vitamin B12, and fortified cereals typically provide ample vitamin B12. It is reassuring that the body stores extra B-12 in the liver (it is the only B-vitamin stored for more than days or weeks). That means you need not ingest yeast or other B-12-rich foods every single day to get the benefits. Another reassuring guideline is that there is no known "upper intake level" or high dose for B-12 so there is no harm in getting more than your body may need.

As with most food items, consumers have a choice of brands and styles so it is a good idea to try more than one kind to decide which tastes best and which is easiest for you to use. Don't just try one brand, decide it tastes funny, then give up! The best bet for most people is probably the flaked variety which has a yellow or golden color from its riboflavin content and can deliciously enhance the flavor (not to mention the nutritional content) of many foods. Following are some sample recipes. Many more can be found on various websites.

SOY-YEAST OMELETS

1 and 1/4 cups water
1 cup yeast flakes
1 cup soy flour (or whole wheat or unbleached)
½ tsp. salt (or vegetable seasoning or mineral salt)
Pinch of garlic or other seasoning (optional)

Mix dry ingredients, Add water and stir to make smooth batter. Pour, like pancakes, onto hot oiled griddle (cold-pressed oils are recommended—see Nutritional Tips chapter). Fill one side of the omelet with diced onions, green peppers, spinach, mushrooms or whatever else you fancy. Flip when edges start to get crisp and the omelet can be easily turned. Fold in half and brown on both sides. Yields 4 – 5 omelets.

GOLDEN GRAVY

½ cup yeast flakes   2 -3 tsp. soy sauce
¼ cup flour   seasoning to taste
1/3 cup oil   water

Toast yeast and flour until you can smell the aromas. Add oil and stir while mixture bubbles and turns golden brown. Add water, still stirring, until it changes to gravy consistency. Stir in soy sauce (or mineral bouillon) and seasonings. Good on mashed potatoes, etc.

ROBERTA'S GOOD SOUP

Sauté 1 medium onion (diced) in 3 T oil. Add:
5 cups boiling water
1 T mineral salt
¼ tsp. celery seed
1 tsp. soy sauce
½ cup nutritional yeast flakes
1½ T soy margarine
2 cups cooked noodles or 1 to 1 ½ cups cooked rice
Simmer 5 minutes. Serve with sprouts and /or crackers.

MACARONI AND 'CHEESE' CASSEROLE

Cook 3½ cups elbow macaroni (many vegetable and whole grain versions are available).

In saucepan, melt ½ cup soy margarine over low heat.

Beat in ½ cup flour with wire whisk until mix (called a 'roux') is smooth and bubbly.

Whip in 3½ cups boiling water, 1½ tsp. mineral salt, 2 T soy sauce, 1½ tsp. garlic powder (or other seasoning), and a pinch of turmeric, beating well to dissolve the roux.

Cook until sauce thickens and bubbles. Then whip in ¼ cup oil and 1 cup nutritional yeast flakes.

Mix part of the sauce with the noodles and place in casserole dish, then pour a generous amount of sauce on top. Sprinkle with paprika and BAKE for 15 minutes in a 350 degree oven. Put under broiler for a few minutes until 'cheese' sauce gets stretchy and crisp.

Serves 5

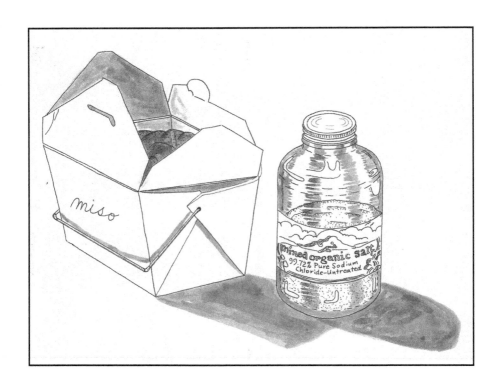

Minerals

Minerals are miniscule inorganic compounds which assist in proper body functioning. Many ailments which might be classified as disease symptoms (that is, in the medical sense or definition of disease, rather than the more illuminating idea of dis-ease of the body due to dietary or other imbalance) may actually be due to a mineral deficiency.

Four percent (4%) of the body's weight is comprised of 60 different minerals, including gold and silver. Vitamins and minerals link together in performing essential tasks in the body. There are 21 minerals considered essential for human nutrition, classified in two categories according to their quantities in the body. Those found in relatively high quantities are termed "macro-minerals" and include calcium, phosphorus, potassium, sulfur, sodium, chloride and magnesium. Minerals which comprise less than 50 parts per million of body weight are called "micro-minerals" or trace elements, such as iron, zinc, selenium, manganese, copper and iodine (see charts below).

Minerals play a role in acid-alkaline balance, nerve impulses, muscle contraction, growth and other processes. They help maintain normal osmotic pressure necessary to move nutrients through cell membranes. That is why, for example, excess sodium intake will cause blood pressure to rise. Following are charts of key minerals with a summary of their functions and some vegetarian dietary sources. Deficiency symptoms are listed unless they are rare or self-explanatory. Ask yourself as you look them over how many of these foods form a regular part of your diet.

Macro-minerals		
Mineral	**Function**	**Sources**
Sodium	Needed for proper fluid balance, nerve transmission, and muscle contraction *Deficiency* is rare in our society	Table salt, soy sauce; large amounts in processed foods; small amounts in breads and vegetables
Chloride	Needed for proper fluid balance, stomach acid	Same sources as for sodium
Potassium	Needed for proper fluid balance, nerve transmission, and muscle contraction *Deficiency*: high blood pressure, constipation, low blood sugar	Fresh fruits and vegetables, whole grains, legumes
Calcium	Important for healthy bones and teeth; helps muscles relax and contract; important in nerve functioning, blood clotting, blood pressure regulation, immune system health	Tofu, tempeh and soy milk; greens (broccoli, mustard greens); legumes; oranges, blackberries
Phosphorus	Important for healthy bones and teeth; found in every cell; part of the system that maintains acid-base balance	Beans, seeds, nuts, oats, quinoa, millet and other grains
Magnesium	Found in bones; needed for making protein, muscle contraction, nerve transmission, immune system health	Nuts and seeds; legumes; leafy, green vegetables; chocolate; artichokes; 'hard' drinking water
Sulfur	Synthesis of antioxidants; hair health; taurine production for cardiovascular system, muscles and central nervous system	Legumes, nuts, kale, Brussels sprouts, broccoli, cabbage onions, asparagus and garlic

Trace minerals		
Mineral	Function	Sources
Iron	Part of the hemoglobin molecule found in red blood cells that carries oxygen in the body; needed for energy metabolism *Deficiency*: anemia, shortness of breath, low sexual interest	Legumes; dried fruits, leafy greens, sea vegetables, iron-enriched breads and cereals
Zinc	Needed for making protein and genetic material; functions in taste perception, wound healing, normal fetal development, production of sperm, normal growth and sexual maturation, immune system health	Legumes, nuts, seeds, oatmeal, broccoli, miso
Iodine	Found in thyroid hormone, which helps regulate growth, development, and metabolism *Deficiency*: hypothyroidism	Baked potatoes, seaweed, iodized salt, prunes, strawberries, green beans
Selenium	Thyroid health; supports immune system, antioxidant *Deficiency*: weakened muscles, premature aging, liver problems	Brazil nuts, pinto beans, brown rice, seeds, green vegetables
Copper	Part of many enzymes; needed for iron metabolism *Deficiency*: anemia, graying and hair loss, heart damage	Legumes, nuts and seeds, whole grains, drinking water
Manganese	Part of many enzymes; involved in metabolism, bone development, wound healing	Nuts, seeds, whole wheat bread, tofu, spinach, kale, black tea

Fluoride	Involved in formation of bones and teeth; helps prevent tooth decay [Note: While some regard fluoride as harmful, extensive scientific research has uncovered no evidence of increased risks of diseases]	Drinking water (either fluoridated or naturally containing fluoride), and most teas
Chromium	Works closely with insulin to regulate blood sugar (glucose) levels	Potatoes, brewer's yeast, whole grains, nuts. broccoli, tomatoes
Molybdenum	Part of some enzymes that help the body use carbohydrates, fats and proteins	Legumes, breads and grains, leafy green vegetables, strawberries

One general concern with getting adequate minerals is soil deficiency. Aggressive farming practices and the use of artificial fertilizers and pesticides result in farmed food that is increasingly deficient in natural minerals. Therefore even frequently eating foods listed here as mineral-rich may not completely ensure you against deficiencies. It is important to get the best quality foods possible from good soil, organic when possible. Supplements can help, provided they also allow for proper absorption of minerals. For example, zinc absorption will be aided by also taking vitamin D; calcium and magnesium are best taken together. You can research how best to take supplements for any suspected deficiency. Spectrographic analysis of hair will give you an individual readout of your absorption of minerals and is capable of identifying as many as 40 trace elements.

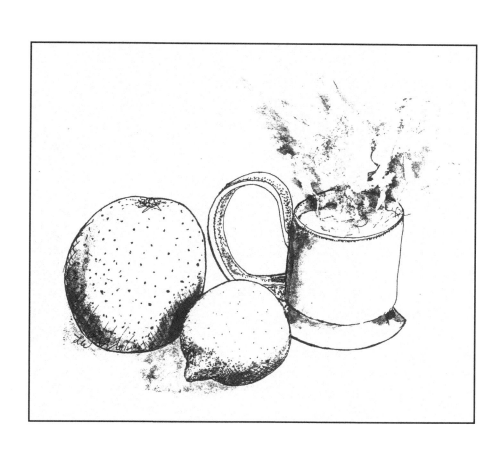

Nutritional Tips

Here are some helpful hints in no particular order or arrangement, but each has proven valuable over the course of time, in some cases going back to ancient yogic practices.

Water

People living in the U. S. are indeed fortunate that we enjoy, in general, clean drinking water. Certainly flavor may vary depending on mineral content, chlorine and other factors. Also some people may unfortunately find themselves living in the vicinity of a fracking site or, if on a well, might well worry about pollution of groundwater from agricultural runoff and/or animal feedlot operations.

Many people have allowed themselves to be convinced that they need to buy bottled "spring" water, which may or may not be what they think they are paying for. The bottled water industry built up a head of steam in the 1980s, and at this point is the second most popular commercial beverage in the U. S., with about half the sales of soft drinks. However, the Natural Resources Defense Council reports that up to 40% pf bottled water is actually filtered tap water. That means that customers are paying more per gallon than the cost of gasoline for water of no better quality than what they could drink for pennies a gallon from their own tap. In fact, it is likely worse since health inspection standards for city (tap) water are many times more stringent than for bottled water.

Then there are the plastic bottles in which the water is sold. Among the chemicals used to produce the bottles, two are of particular concern:

Bisphenol A (BPA) may cause cancer in people, as reported on breast cancer awareness websites, because its estrogen-like activity makes it a hormone disruptor.

Just as worrisome are *phthalates*, which have been linked to abnormal male sexual development, male infertility, premature breast development, cancer, miscarriage, premature birth and asthma. Because phthalates are not chemically bound to the plastic polymer, they can easily migrate out.

Think about how long the water may have been in the plastic bottle before you drink it, and it is unlikely it has been kept refrigerated. Both heat and time result in leaching of chemicals from the plastic and growth of bacteria in the water, since few bottled waters are sold with a sterile seal, such as you might find on eye drops sold at the drug store. So no matter what quality the water originally may have been, once it is bottled it is almost certainly compromised. The best advice for your health (and your budget!) is to forget about buying water in plastic bottles, and filter your own tap water. You can buy an inexpensive filter pitcher, or for a couple hundred dollars install an under-sink reverse-osmosis filtering system.

Carry your own glass, steel, or ceramic water bottle filled with filtered tap water.

Lemon juice

Upon arising, a mixture of hot water and fresh-squeezed lemon juice will prove beneficial in controlling appetite and cleansing the digestive system, as well as aiding regularity. You can sweeten with honey, fructose, or simply squeeze juice from half and orange into the mix. Limes are a good substitute if lemons are hard to find or costly. This tip is recommended in numerous health books, by yoga instructors and even by coaches for modelling and other pursuits in which health and healthy appearance are valued.

You don't need much lemon juice to enjoy this beverage; just be sure to dilute it so that you are not bathing your teeth in straight lemon juice. Actually lemon juice becomes alkaline when digested by the body, even though, as a citrus fruit, it has acidic quality outside the body. So if a person sucks on fresh lemons or limes all the time such a practice could damage tooth enamel. But drinking lemon-water does not expose the teeth for excessive amounts of time to high citrus acidic levels in the mouth, thereby causing no harm to the enamel. In fact, it can improve plaque-stained teeth and bad breath. Drinking diluted lemon juice in the morning has been an Ayurvedic practice for a long time; Ayurvedic medicine is a system of Hindu traditional medicine of Vedic tradition.

Nasal Rinse

While this topic isn't about something to either ingest or to avoid, assuming that better health is the goal for studying nutrition, this tip can work wonders. After all, the very air we breathe plays an important role in good health; it is a cliché that getting fresh air will do you good. Besides moving to the seashore, the mountains, or next to a waterfall, one thing that is easy to do is to make sure your nasal passages are not obstructed so that your lungs can get the oxygen you need. Here is a statement from WebMD:

> Nasal irrigation involves flushing out the nose and sinuses with salt water (saline). It is done using a variety of methods including application with a bulb syringe or using a 'neti pot.' Neti pots are used by practitioners of yoga and Ayurvedic medicine. The neti pots look like small teapots. They are filled with saline solution and poured through the nostrils. No method of nasal irrigation has been consistently shown to work better than another.
>
> Saline irrigation flushes out mucus and irritants from the sinuses, improves the flow of air through the nose, and reduces nasal swelling. It is also used to treat sinus infections, allergies, the common cold, post-nasal drip, and other conditions affecting the nose.
>
> *(http://www.webmd.com/vitamins-supplements/*
> *ingredientmono-1229-nasal%20irrigation)*

I have done nasal irrigation every morning for many years and it has become a routine, just like brushing teeth. You don't even need any special equipment. Simply sprinkle some sea salt into a half-cup of warm water, pour some into the cupped palm of your hand and sniff in some of the saline solution. Give it a few seconds, then "exhale" it as if blowing your nose into the sink. Repeat two or three times to give the nasal passages a good irrigation. I am so used to clear breathing that on the rare day I forget to do this routine, my nose feels comparatively stuffed up and my breathing feels obstructed.

Should you think you are going to drown yourself by attempting this, there is little risk. Ocean swimming gives the same effect; you usually get salt water in your mouth and nose, but far from drowning or choking you just sniff it out and usually feel refreshed and cleaner. The practice is an important part of the yogic system of body cleansing techniques that is associated with Hinduism, and has been practiced for thousands of years. Yogis believe that it not only helps to avoid respiratory illnesses, but since yoga practice includes attention to breathing, gives spiritual benefits as well.

Shampoos and soaps

Choosing body cleansers and cosmetics is part of a larger issue of chemicals in cosmetics. It is an important health issue which gets little publicity. For example, most commercial shampoos contain *sodium lauryl or laureth sulfate* (SLS), presumably because it is the cheapest ingredient to get the foaming effect that consumer associate with clean hair (though natural surfactants or foaming agents will get your hair just as clean even if they don't foam as much). Unfortunately SLS is a harsh chemical also used as an engine degreaser, and at the very least strips hair of essential oils it needs to stay healthy, breaks down protein and interferes with healthy hair growth. Fortunately there are shampoos that are SLS-free, though you much more likely to find a selection of them in health stores than in drug stores and supermarkets. Surprisingly, SLS is an ingredient even in more expensive and 'salon' shampoos, so spending more for supposed 'quality' products is no substitute for reading the ingredients on the label. While you might assume that the Food and Drug Administration will protect consumers, since body care and cosmetic products are not considered medicines, they are not subject to FDA approval, and the FDA does not regulate the body care industry unless it receives mass complaints about a product's safety.

An even more alarming common shampoo ingredient is *phthalates*, used both as gelling agents and to make fragrance last longer. Phthalates are known endocrine disruptors, with a chemical structure that mimics human hormones. Exposure to high levels of phthalates during pregnancy can lead to birth defects, specifically linked to male children's genitals and reproductive systems. Among other negative effects, phthalates can promote obesity. The European Union and Canada enacted strict regulations on the use of phthalates, but U. S. regulation is comparatively lax. In fact the EU bans a long list of chemicals that are still permitted in cosmetic formulas in the U. S., so it is a case of "buyer beware."

Here is a brief list of other potentially toxic shampoo ingredients (also found in other personal care items):

Dioxane, a known carcinogen

Diethanolamine or DEA which reacts with nitrites to form NDEA, a dangerous carcinogen

Propylene Glycol which is also used in engine coolants and antifreeze, paints, adhesives, enamels and varnishes as a solvent or surfactant

Parabens; the EPA has linked methyl parabens in particular to metabolic, developmental, hormonal, and neurological disorders, as well as to various cancers

Artificial fragrances, which can contain hundreds—even thousands—of chemicals

The Environmental Working Group's *Skin Deep Cosmetic Safety Database* is an excellent resource to help you find safe natural personal care products. A newer site called *Good Guide* is also helpful in finding and evaluating healthful, green products. Some simple advice is that if some ingredient is hard to pronounce or wouldn't seem safe to eat, don't buy it. Choose shampoos and other cosmetics that clearly state on the label, "Not tested on animals." The reason products are tested on animals in the first place is that they contain toxic ingredients that may cause harm to humans. Lastly, don't be fooled by the idea that toxic ingredients are present in small amounts. Lots of people use up to 20 cosmetics and cleaners daily. While women typically use more, men also use shampoos and other hair products, deodorants, colognes, shaving creams, toothpaste, mouthwash, soaps and tanning lotions. It is a worthwhile and even vital investment in the health of your scalp, skin and general health to avoid products with toxic ingredients and invest in safe alternatives.

There is also discussion of cosmetics in the Externals chapter; if some information is repeated there it is to increase the likelihood that readers just dipping into selected chapters will come across this important topic.

Vegetable oils

Udo Erasmus, author of the book *Fats That Heal, Fats That Kill*, writes that, "Cooking oils are highly processed, using manufacturing methods that are destructive to oil molecules. These practices are utilized primarily to lengthen and stabilize the shelf life of oils. After oils are pressed or solvent extracted from seeds and nuts, they are degummed, refined, bleached, and deodorized. The result is known as an *RBD* (refined, bleached, deodorized) and these oils, as a result, become colorless, odorless, and tasteless." *(http://www.udoerasmus. com/articles/udo/bbaco.htm)*

Most oils go rancid when temperatures exceed 125 degrees, so that the European standard for pressing them is to keep temperatures below 122 degrees. Rancid oils harm cells and use up precious antioxidants. The commercial degumming process treats oils with water heated to high temperatures between 188 and 206 degrees Fahrenheit. And since such processing results in rancidity, giving oils an unpleasant smell, they are deodorized by passing steam over hot oil in a vacuum at between 440 and 485 degrees Fahrenheit.

Oils that are best for quality and health rather than shelf life will be:

- Pressed from organically grown seeds and nuts. Most corn and canola oil is genetically modified but organic certification generally guarantees that it is not.
- Protected from light, air, and heat during pressing, filtering, and filling.
- Sold in dark glass bottles that say unrefined on the label. Unrefined is better for health and quality but tends to go rancid more quickly.

- Look for *expeller pressed* oils by manufacturers that keep the pressing temperature low. The expeller pressure temperature may be listed on the label. Look for pressing temperatures below 122 degrees Fahrenheit.
- Oils made to these standards are safe and desirable but are not to be used for cooking!

Heat tolerant oils that are best to use for cooking will be:

- Coconut oil
- Palm kernel oil
- Palm oil
- Cacao oil
- Shea nut oil

Olive oil can be cold-pressed, but is not recommended for frying or high heat cooking because the heat will damage the oil, which can instead be added after cooking. Olive oil can be stored at room temperature, though a cool cupboard is preferable to the stove top. Another method is to put olive oil you will readily use in a small container and keep the rest in the refrigerator for later use. Refrigerated olive oil will solidify and turn cloudy, but returning it to room temperature restores its fluidity and color. Refrigeration is best for long-term storage of all olive oils except premium extra-virgin ones.

So to sum up, the best vegetable oils will be expeller-pressed, organic, and unrefined with no hydrogenated fats. Whenever possible buy oils in opaque containers to keep out light, and *store them in the refrigerator.* Never store out on the counter where the oil is exposed to light.

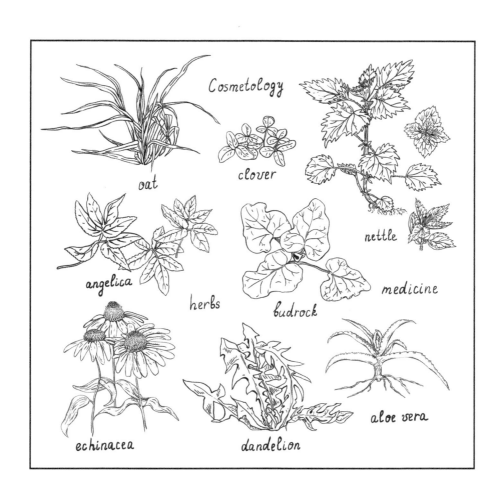

Cosmetology

oat

clover

nettle

angelica

herbs

budrock

medicine

echinacea

dandelion

aloe vera

Seasonings

In our modern world with increasingly cheap, high calorie food (example, fast food — or "junk food"), prepared foods that are high in things like salt, sugars or fat, combined with our increasingly sedentary lifestyles, increasing urbanization and changing modes of transportation, it is no wonder that obesity has rapidly increased in the last few decades, around the world.

--Anup Shah, *Obesity*, Global Issues.org,
November 21, 2010

Inorganic salt is not a food; it is not utilized by the body. Some of it is retained, causing stiffening of the joints, arthritis, hardening of the arteries and kidney disease…In a high enough concentration it inhibits cell metabolism, eventually causing death of the cells. To reduce the concentration of salt, your body will retain an excess of water in the tissues.

--Victoras Kulvinskas, *Survival into the 21ˢᵗ Century*

Our standard American diet encourages us to drown out the natural flavors of food under a blanket of salt, catsup, mustard, bottled sauces and condiments. When it comes to processed foods this hyper-flavoring also includes monosodium glutamate (MSG) and artificial flavors. Companies and labs specialize in creating flavors that mimic almost anything food manufacturers request. More than 3000 additives and preservatives can be found in processed foods. They are all synthesized chemicals that don't even have common names. Most artificial flavorings are derived from petroleum and contain many chemical ingredients; most have not been studied for safety or toxicity, partly since food processors claim they are added in 'trace amounts.' Dr. David Kessler, former FDA Commissioner, addressed the issue on a *60 Minutes* broadcast, questioning whether all these flavorings are really food. "We're living in a food carnival, these flavors are so stimulating they hijack our brain," he asserts. (*A Natural and Artificial Flavoring Factory*, Huffington Post, September 13, 2015)

These flavorings and condiments can be addictive as well, especially sugar, salt and artificial sweeteners. Researchers claim that salt is addictive in the same way as cigarettes or hard drugs, inducing a craving triggering the same genes, brain cells and brain connections. Professor Derek Denton, of the University of Melbourne, says of the research, "We have demonstrated that one classic instinct, the hunger for salt, is providing neural organization that subserves addiction to opiates and cocaine." (Duke University Medical Center, *Science Daily*, "Salt Appetite is Linked to drug Addiction," July 29, 2011)

According to information by the Global Healing Center, commercial table salt, sold at supermarkets or found on the table of your favorite restaurant, unlike naturally harvested sea salt or Himalayan salt, is created by taking natural salt (or crude oil flake leftovers) and cooking it at 1200° Fahrenheit. When unprocessed salt is heated up to this temperature, it starts to lose most of its eighty important naturally occurring elements. Then come additives: sodium solo-co-aluminate, iodide, sodium bicarbonate, fluoride, anti-caking agents, toxic amounts of potassium iodide and aluminum derivatives. MSG and/or white processed sugar are added to help stabilize the iodine. And then it is colored white with bleach. Much of it is the actual flaky residue from oil digging; crude oil extract is one way we produce table salt.

Clearly the wise choice for salt is natural, sun-dried sea salt or Himalayan mined salt. Even with these healthier choices you don't want to overdo it. Our processed foods are loaded with salt, as are canned soups and common condiments. In American society it would be difficult to get too little salt. Better food choices can help people avoid overdoing the salt. Eating celery, seaweed, raw cultured vegetables, Swiss chard, or spinach will provide extra sodium when cravings strike.

The goal should be to wean ourselves off of these concentrated flavorings and learn to appreciate the more subtle and natural flavors of the foods we have buried underneath them. A plain baked potato can taste satisfying all by itself, and need not be slathered in condiments. Following are healthier choices to flavor foods that provide additional health benefits.

DULSE or sea kelp, available inexpensively in bulk powder or flakes, provides iodine and other minerals such potassium and calcium and is a good transitional substitute for salt and pepper (though pepper in moderation presents no health challenges and can even be beneficial).

VEGIT or other powdered mixes made from dehydrated vegetables are great substitute seasonings, but be sure to read the label since some of these still include salt.

LIQUID AMINOS (Bragg brand is one) derived from soy protein, with no added salt, can be used as a substitute for soy sauce.

MINERAL BOULLION (Bernard Jensen in one brand) can also be used in place of soy sauce.

HERBS can be grown indoors or out or purchased in bulk and used in many ways with food. They can provide a great spectrum of truly natural flavors.

NUTRITIONAL YEAST (see Yeast chapter) not only provides great nutrition, but can give a nutty, cheesy flavor to foods. Try it as a substitute for processed Parmesan cheese, for example.

MISO can be used as a flavoring in many ways. It does contain salt, but yields a lot of flavor in quite small amounts, and is high in lactobacillus, acidophilus, protein and minerals (see Fermented Foods chapter for more on miso).

APPLE CIDER VINEGAR is made by fermenting pressed apple juice until the sugars turn to vinegar. It should be made from organic apples and should be unheated, unfiltered and unpasteurized to keep the 'mother' intact. The 'mother' consists of strands of proteins, enzymes and friendly bacteria. This healthful vinegar can prove to be a versatile flavoring and many swear by its health benefits.

Natural spices will lose flavor and color during long storage so should be purchased in quantities which you will readily use. Many health-oriented stores sell herbs and spices in bulk which allows consumers to purchase as little or as much as they wish. Spices and herbs keep best in a cool, dry place in air-tight containers. Heat hastens flavor loss and moisture can cause caking, color change and infestation. You might save small bottles from commercial spices to use to store your own bulk purchases. Be sure containers are tightly sealed after each use so that volatile oils are not lost. Spices will keep good aroma and flavor for up to six months, but after that should be replaced. Exceptions are whole spices (nutmeg, cloves, vanilla beans, etc.) which keep flavor indefinitely.

Growing fresh herbs and grinding your own whole spices are worth doing for best flavor and full benefits of the plants. Try, for example, fresh basil leaves cut up in homemade tomato soup. Flavor will be much fuller and subtler then when using dry basil leaves as commonly sold. Using a fresh vanilla bean yields a similar surprise in flavor. If dried parsley flakes are all you've ever experienced, buy some fresh parsley, which in addition to enhancing flavor and appearance of foods, is an herbal blood purifier. Parsley is a healthy habit in salads, soups and vegetable dishes. You can experiment with cilantro too, which goes particularly well with Mexican foods.

Ground spices add flavor readily and can be added 10 to 15 minutes before a dish is done cooking, or simply crumble fresh onto salads or other vegetables. Whole spices can be used for longer-cooking dishes in which simmering will extract full flavor and aroma. Tied in a cheesecloth bag, they are easily removed. Herbs, whole or in leaves, should be crumbled just before use to release flavor. Seeds will be more flavorful if toasted.

You will acquire your own favorites by experimenting with herbs and spices in your food preparation. Many alternative seasoning mixes can be found on the shelves of your local health store. Just be sure to read the labels and avoid those with salt listed as a primary ingredient (typically labels list ingredients by amount included, starting with those with the largest share in the mix). By turning to the wealth of herbs, spices and alternative flavorings you can leave behind the 'chemical carnival' of commercial condiments, and even better, learn to appreciate the true flavors of food as nature intended.

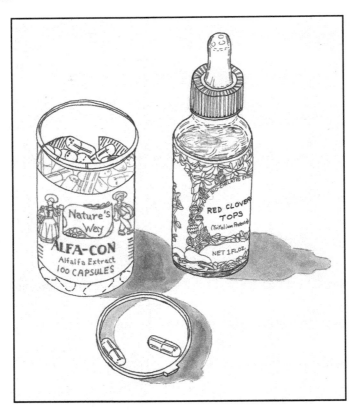

VITAMINS AND HERBS

Research has emerged since the first edition of this book which casts into doubt the usefulness of taking supplemental vitamins. A quick cruise of the internet will yield the results of massive studies that demonstrate negligible benefits from taking multivitamins. Here's one sample from WebMD:

> A research review assessed the evidence from 27 studies on vitamin and mineral supplements that included more than 450,000 people. That study, conducted for the U.S. Preventive Services Task Force, found no evidence that supplements offer a benefit for heart disease or that they delay death from any cause. They found only a minimal benefit for cancer risk. (WebMD, *Vitamins and Supplements*)

The bottom line is that the best way to get the vitamins and minerals your body needs is to eat healthful foods. Something like 40% of Americans are taking multivitamins, and overall half of Americans take some kind of supplement, but trying to use vitamins as 'insurance' while eating lots of processed food, fast food and junk food simply will not help. The money spent on vitamins would be much better spent on healthful foods, especially fresh fruits and vegetables full of vitamins, minerals and nutrients.

It is instructive to note that dietary supplements are not regulated by the U.S. Food and Drug Administration in the same way as prescription drugs are. Manufacturers do not have to prove safety or effectiveness. An additional factor is that many raw ingredients for supplements are shipped from China, but the FDA has not inspected any of the factories there. As a result, supplements may be contaminated with heavy metals, pesticides, or prescription drugs, according to Consumer Reports and other consumer advocacy groups. And though it is against the law for companies to claim that any supplements can prevent, treat, or cure disease, nevertheless unethical marketing may lead consumers to believe they can.

Consumer Reports warns specifically against a dozen supplements they consider especially hazardous: aconite, bitter orange, chaparral, colloidal silver, coltsfoot, comfrey, country mallow, germanium, greater celandine, kava, lobelia, and yohimbe. The FDA has issued warnings concerning at least eight of them as long ago as 1993.

The good news is that some supplements CAN improve health, including calcium, cranberry extract, fish oil, glucosamine sulfate, lactase (if drinking milk!!), lactobacillus, psyllium, pigeum, SAMe, St. John's wart and vitamin D. Also vitamin C and vitamin E oils can be added to this list and will be discussed below the following chart which details some of these:

NAME	BENEFITS	SIDE EFFECTS	INTERACTIONS
CALCIUM (calcium carbonate, calcium citrate, calcium gluconate)	Take with vitamin D for preventing and treating bone loss and osteoporosis. Daily dose appears to reduce PMS symptoms.	Belching, gas	May decrease effectiveness of some antibiotics, osteoporosis drugs, and thyroid drugs.

CRANBERRY (American cranberry, large cranberry, cranberry extract)	May help prevent recurrent urinary-tract infections.	May cause upset stomach or diarrhea in large amounts	Might increase effects of the blood thinner warfarin.
FISH OIL (EPA/DHA, omega-3 fatty acids, PUFA)	Reduces triglyceride levels. May decrease risk of heart attack, stroke, and further hardening of the arteries in people with heart disease.	Fishy aftertaste, upset stomach, nausea, loose stools. High doses can increase levels of LDL (bad) cholesterol in some people	May increase effect of blood-thinning drugs and high blood pressure medications.
GLUCOSAMINE SULFATE (G6S, glucosamine sulfate 2KCl, glucosamine sulfate-potassium chloride)	Treatment for reducing symptoms of osteoarthritis of the knee. May slow progression of osteoarthritis.	Nausea, heartburn, diarrhea, headache, constipation	May increase the blood-thinning effect of warfarin and cause bruising and bleeding.
LACTASE (beta-galactosidase)	Reduces gastrointestinal symptoms in lactose intolerant people when added to milk.	No reported side effects	None known. *See "Dairy" chapter of this book for discussion of health risks of drinking milk.*
LACTOBACILLUS (acidophilus, acidophilus lactobacillus, probiotics)	May help prevent diarrhea while taking antibiotics. *See "Fermented Foods" chapter for more health benefits.*	Gas. People with poor immune function should check with their doctor first	Might cause infection in people taking immunosuppressant drugs.
PSYLLIUM (blond plantago, blonde psyllium, plantago, isabgola)	Effective as a bulk laxative for relieving constipation. May lower cholesterol in people with mild to moderately high cholesterol.	Gas, stomach pain, diarrhea, constipation, nausea. Some people can have a serious allergic response that requires immediate medical attention	Might decrease effectiveness of carbamazepine, an antiseizure drug; digoxin, a heart drug; and lithium, for bipolar disorder. May cause low blood sugar if taken with some diabetes drugs.

PYGEUM (African plum tree, African prune)	Likely effective for reducing symptoms of an enlarged prostate.	Nausea, abdominal pain	None known.
SAMe (ademetionine, adenosylmethionine, S-Adenosyl-L-Methionine, sammy)	Helpful in reducing symptoms of major depression, reducing pain, and improving functioning in people with osteoarthritis.	GI symptoms, dry mouth, headache, mild insomnia, anorexia, sweating, dizziness, anxiety, and nervousness	Possible toxic reaction if taken with the cough suppressant dextromethorphan, certain antidepressants, or narcotic pain relievers.
ST. JOHN'S WORT (Hypericum perforatum, Saynt Johannes Wort, SJW)	Helpful for improving symptoms of some forms of depression.	Insomnia, vivid dreams, anxiety, dizziness, headache, skin rash, and tingling. Can cause sun-sensitive skin	Can decrease the effectiveness of birth-control pills, heart medications, HIV/AIDS drugs, and warfarin. Might also increase the effects or side effects of certain antidepressants.
VITAMIN D (Cholecalciferol, vitamin D3, ergocalciferol, vitamin D2)	Take with calcium to help prevent osteoporosis. Might help reduce bone loss in people taking corticosteroids.	Rare, though extreme amounts might cause weakness, fatigue, headache, and nausea.	Might reduce the effectiveness of some medications, such as atorvastatin (Lipitor), other heart medications, birth-control pills, HIV/AIDS drugs.

Based on information from Natural Medicines Comprehensive Database, Professional Version, June 2010

Vitamin C, so strongly championed by Nobel Prize winner Linus Pauling, can be effective against stress, skin aging, symptoms of common colds, and risk of stroke if formulated from rosehips. There is no known overdose of vitamin C since the body excretes what it can't use. Some health experts argue that the natural citrus bioflavonoids in fresh fruit make for more effective absorption.

Vitamin E oil, particularly if taken together with vitamin C, can be beneficial in protecting against toxins from air pollution, in relieving symptoms of premenstrual syndrome, eye disorders such as cataracts, neurological diseases such as Alzheimer's and diabetes. Its antioxidant properties can boost the immune system. It is also recommended as a topical supplement for the skin, both as a moisturizer and even to treat scars and acne.

HERBS are the original and natural 'pharmaceuticals' used, for example, in China for a thousand years before the advent of modern pharmacy. Other countries with a similarly long history of herbal remedies are India and Japan. In ancient Egypt pharmacological knowledge was recorded in papyri dating back to 1550 B.C., and ancient Greece developed a group of experts in medicinal plants during and after the time of Hippocrates.

Chinese herbal medicine in particular employs a holistic approach, focusing on health and prevention rather than the 'disease intervention' strategy typical of modern Western medicine. Basically, herbs are used instead of or in place of pharmaceutical medicines, as general nerve and body tonics, as preventatives against disease, or for both tonic and enjoyment, as with herbal teas. They can be taken to alleviate symptoms of particular diseases as well. They can also be applied locally for injuries when made into salves, oils, plasters and so forth.

While this chapter will sample some herbs and their applications, there are entire books dedicated to cataloguing herbs and their uses. One classic is Jethro Kloss' *Back to Eden,* in which the author lists many common herbs by name (giving descriptions, properties and usage as well as folklore) along with a section that matches ailments with their recommended herbal cures. Another good reference is Rodale's *Illustrated Encyclopedia of Herbs,* listing 140 herbs including history, uses and cultivation and is fully illustrated with drawings and color photos. Of course there are many more excellent guides to be found.

While we may be tempted to think of using herbs as 'granny cures' or 'folk medicine,' remember that pharmaceutical medicine has been with us an infinitesimal length of time (really just the last 100 years dating back to the passage of the Pure food and Drug Act in 1906) compared to age-old remedies based on indigenous flora. One personal story concerns a time when from swimming in polluted waters I got a serious and persistent eye infection. A doctor gave me a prescription, but it seemed to be of no help in curing the infection. Out of frustration I tried using the herb *eyebright.* My eye infection cleared quickly, and when I returned for a follow-up my doctor, seeing the infection was gone, took careful notes when I told him about using eyebright so that he could recommend it to future patients with eye infections—the sign of an open-minded practitioner. Lest people might suspect that my eye healed itself or that my cure was psychosomatic, scientifically, it is thought that the chemicals in eyebright act as astringents and indeed kill bacteria.

There are several available forms in which to buy herbs. One way is to get seeds and cultivate your own herb garden. Especially for culinary herbs this is a delicious way to season food and to avoid processed and manufactured spices and condiments. Another approach is to purchase either fresh or dried herbs, especially from stores selling them in bulk as many health stores offer. You can purchase empty gelatin capsules and fill them with herbs in powder form. (Since gelatin is not vegetarian and may cause residue in the digestive tract if consumed frequently, an alternative is edible starch paper, or 'potato circles' which can be wrapped around herbs and sealed and can accommodate relatively bulky herb mixes). A more expensive but efficient way to get herbs is to buy them encapsulated or in the form of liquid extracts. Last but not least, some people simply chew on leaves or dried stems of their favorite herbs. While bitter flavor might put off some, anyone can try chewing on culinary herbs such as licorice, cinnamon or vanilla before attempting the more exotic flavors.

Herbs used therapeutically range from single herbs such as sage for colds to groups of herbs combined as 'formulae' for remedies. So, for example, a laxative blend might combine *pumpkin seed, culver's root, may apple, violet leaves, poke root, cascara sagrada, witch hazel bark, mullein, comfrey root* and *slippery elm bark*. The Chinese herbs *foti* and *dong quai, saw palmetto, aloe vera, horsetail, ginkgo biloba* and *stinging nettle* can be used singly or in combination to treat hair loss, regrowth of hair and restoration of hair color. An herbal 'nerve soother' might combine *valerian, chamomile, horsetail grass, passion flower* and *wood betony*.

Some single herbs are associated with particular applications, such as *cassea bark* for circulation or *chervil* for memory and concentration. These two taken together might be recommended for people who do mental labor (such as writers!). Some herbs are regarded as having more general application to health, such as *golden seal,* recommended for eyes, bowel and bladder troubles, catarrhal conditions, throat trouble, sore gums, skin diseases, stomach and liver troubles and even colds.

Another single herb that has become fairly well-known to Americans is ginseng. About ginseng my friend Denis remarked, "Oh yes, I tried that and it didn't work." His joke serves to underscore our default desire for the instant cure rather than a more holistic approach to good health. Ginseng falls under the category "for which no specific nutritional claims are made" meaning that it has not been evaluated by the FDA for safety, effectiveness, or purity. However, it has been used for thousands of years, and unless one proves allergic to it, which is rare, there are no outstanding side effects so long as it is taken in moderate amounts and is not known to have an adverse reaction with other medications taken, so ginseng seems like a safe herb with which to experiment.

According to the University of Maryland Medical Center, "Panax ginseng may help boost the immune system, reduce risk of cancer, and improve mental performance and well-being. Laboratory studies in animals have found that American ginseng is effective in boosting the immune system, and as an antioxidant. Other studies show that American ginseng might have therapeutic potential for…a number of conditions" (*https://umm.edu/health/medical/altmed/herb/asian-ginseng*). Their list includes diabetes, cancer, colds and flu, and attention deficit hyperactivity disorder as well as general immune system enhancement. To this salutary list Chinese tradition adds the ability to instill energy, stamina, libido enhancement, and longevity. Ginseng is available in many forms, including as a bottled liquid extract containing the whole ginseng root. Curiously, a mature root is shaped like a human, earning it the name "Ren Shen" which means "Man Root" in Chinese.

So herbs such as *golden seal* and *ginseng* enter the classification of general tonics that can be used as a matter of regular habit rather than treating them as medicines to be applied in times of particular trouble. In fact that approach applies to the general science of good nutrition as well. Nothing is a miracle cure, and few foods, food supplements, herbs or other nutrients will change any condition overnight. But taken along with exercise, fresh air and other positive practices such as yoga or meditation, such an approach to nutrition and the "science of living" cannot help but return great dividends for health on the initial investment.

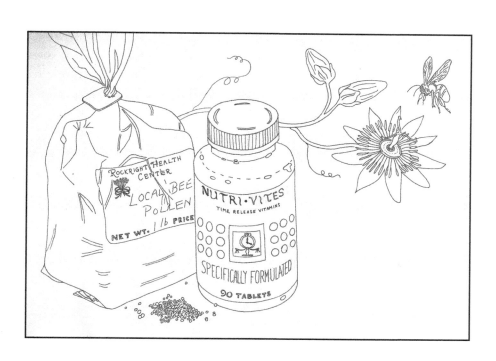

Food Supplements

We have already reviewed how commercial vitamin supplements probably do little to improve your health. The best nutrients come from the foods you consume. But here are some "superfoods" that might yield benefits if you add them to your diet. One category is the green foods such as *wheatgrass* and *spirulina* detailed in a different chapter. Another group is fermented foods such as *miso* and yogurt, discussed in the Fermented Foods chapter. But there are other highly beneficial foods, some perhaps more familiar than others, and some that can be found in optimal formulations.

Wheat Germ

One great food supplement is WHEAT GERM. This is the part of the wheat berry which germinates for the berry to grow into wheat grass. Wheat germ contains 23 nutrients, is high in protein, and contains essential fatty acids including vitamin E. It provides B vitamins, fiber, minerals including iron, zinc, magnesium, calcium, selenium and manganese, and phytosterols which can lower unhealthy cholesterol and promote a healthy heart. But the germ cannot survive long outside the protection of the berry, so to increase shelf life (a familiar motive for processing and preserving foods) manufacturers toast the wheat germ. Some commercial wheat germ is completely defatted so that it can be sold without going rancid for up to a year. Unfortunately, the defatting removes all of the vitamin E. Incidentally, manufacturers of white flour also remove the valuable wheat germ to give longer shelf life to white bread—a great argument for eating whole wheat products.

Clearly raw wheat germ will deliver the most nutrients, even though toasting wheat germ gives it a nutty and appealing flavor. Some packagers lightly toast the germ, though this is something you could do yourself at home. Simply place the raw wheat germ in a heavy skillet and toast over medium heat stirring constantly. Remove from the pan immediately when it is toasted as much as you want. Of course it is unlikely you are going to sit down to a big bowl of wheat germ, so its isolated taste will not be an issue. In any case, raw wheat germ has a pleasant enough flavor as is: slightly nutty, slightly bland. Typical uses are:

- Stir it into yogurt
- Add a tablespoon or two to a smoothie or shake
- Sprinkle it over cereal or cooked oatmeal
- Toss it into a salad
- Sprinkle it on a peanut butter sandwich
- Use it in raw vegan recipes or bake into muffins and casseroles
- Use it for making pancakes or waffles

You can even make a tea out of it by brewing one tablespoon per two cups of water; steep for 20 minutes, then filter and drink.

It is best to buy raw wheat germ either bagged and refrigerated, or vacuum-packed. It will lose nutrients and become rancid quickly when exposed to air. Ideally, at home it should be stored tightly sealed in the freezer for no more than two months. For ease of use I keep a glass jar of raw wheat germ in the refrigerator, ready to mix into or sprinkle onto other foods.

Sunflower Seeds

Another convenient food supplement is sunflower seeds, which, like wheat germ, are most nutritious eaten raw. Sunflower seeds deliver high levels of protein, antioxidants, minerals and linoleic acid (an essential fatty acid). They're an excellent source of vitamin E, dietary fiber, selenium, magnesium, potassium, zinc, phosphorus, vitamin B1, vitamin B6 and folate. A quarter-cup serving provides 90 percent of daily Vitamin E requirements to help prevent asthma, arthritis, colon cancer and cardiovascular disease. Magnesium promotes a healthy immune system and strong bones, potassium improves kidney functioning, and zinc supports healthy overall growth.

Sunflower seeds even make you happy! The kernels contain tryptophan, an amino acid that helps create the neurotransmitter serotonin. In turn, serotonin eases tension, relaxes nerves and prevents depression. And their plentiful supply of selenium gives you a nutrient believed to lighten a mood almost instantaneously.

They make a great addition to breads, cakes, cookies and muffins. To better mix in with flour or stirred into other dishes they can be finely ground. They can be mixed into salads or sprinkled onto hot or cold cereals or into yogurt. They are also a crunchy substitute for bacon bits and croutons on cooked vegetables and salads. As with wheat germ, you can also toast them to bring out their subtle flavor and extend their shelf life, though remember that the more toasting, the greater the loss of delicate nutrients.

As with wheat germ, since sunflower seeds have a high fat content and are prone to rancidity, it is best to store them in an airtight container in the refrigerator. They can also be stored in the freezer without greatly affecting their texture or flavor.

Raw Almonds

Almonds provide a variety of nutrients and antioxidants to help your body thrive. At least nine clinical studies of record show that almonds may have a beneficial impact on heart health and cholesterol. One of the healthiest aspects of almonds appears to be their skins, rich in antioxidants including phenols, flavonoids and phenolic acids.

Unfortunately, in 2007 (due to two incidents of *salmonella* contamination in batches of raw almonds) government agencies mandated that all raw almonds sold in the U. S. be either pasteurized or treated with propylene oxide gas. With pasteurization the almonds are steamed to a temperature of 200 degrees, destroying nutrients in the process. And since propylene oxide is classified by the U.S. Environmental Protection Agency (EPA) as a probable human carcinogen, inevitable residues on nuts is problematic. If producers' regular manufacturing includes either dry roasting or blanching to achieve the same risk reduction, then they are excused from the mandated treatments. If the almonds are sold as *organic* they will not be gassed.

So to get the most out of eating almonds, seek truly raw, organic almonds that have not been pasteurized. One option is to buy from a grower at a local farmer's market, because farmers are granted an exemption if selling their almonds directly to customers at local markets. Another is to order online from a certified organic almond grower outside of the United States who exports almonds to this country.

In addition to the usual ways you might use almonds, you can chop them up to add texture and flavor to plain yogurt, slice them onto salads and sautéed vegetables, or add some almond butter to a breakfast shake. To roast almonds at home, do so gently in a 160-170°F oven for 15-20 minutes to preserve the healthy oils. Blanching nuts removes their skin so that they are no longer considered a whole food.

Chia seeds

These are the same seeds from the infamous "Chia Pets" that were a fad some years back, though people who bought the sprouting Pets may not have realized how nutritious chia seeds can be. Native to South America, chia seeds were an important food for the Aztecs and Mayans. They deliver protein, fiber, B-vitamins, Omega-3 fatty acids, zinc and other minerals. Chia seeds are a "whole grain" food, usually grown organically, non-GMO and naturally free of gluten.

They are rich in natural anti-oxidants and provide 14% protein by weight. Since they absorb 10 or 12 times their weight in water they expand in the stomach, which should increase the feeling of fullness and slow the absorption of food. So those interested in weight loss may benefit from chia seeds. They are high in several nutrients important for bone health, including calcium, phosphorus, and magnesium. Their higher calcium content by weight than dairy products makes them a great source of calcium for people who don't eat dairy. Research has indicated that chia seeds may be helpful in improving conditions of type 2 diabetes.

Chia seeds are a versatile food supplement. They can be eaten raw, soaked in juice, or added to porridges, puddings, and baked goods. You can also sprinkle them on top of cereal, yogurt, vegetables or rice dishes. Since they readily absorb both water and fat, they can be used to thicken sauces and even used in recipes as an egg substitute. Two or three tablespoons per day, or about 20 grams, provide an adequate dosage of chia seeds.

Marmite

In the late 19th Century the German scientist Justus Liebig discovered that brewer's yeast could be concentrated, bottled and eaten. The Marmite Food Company was founded in 1902 in Burton-on-Trent, Staffordshire, England, using raw material readily available from the town's brewers. Production uses yeast residue left over from the beer brewing process. The yeast is specially treated, mixed with salt, vegetable extracts, vitamins (including B12, which is especially welcome for vegetarians) and other proprietary ingredients. It is considered so beneficial that it was made a part of British soldiers' ration packs in both world wars. An English scientist found that the folic acid in Marmite could be used to treat anemia and it was used to treat malnutrition in workers in India during a malaria epidemic in the 1930s. Similar food products are *Vegemite*, produced in Australia and New Zealand, the Swiss *Cenovis* and the German *Vitam-R*.

Marmite is very low in sugar, low in calories, contains no saturated fat and is completely vegetarian. A 4-gram serving provides 36 percent of the recommended daily allowance of vitamin B3, 50 percent of the RDA for folic acid and 17 per cent of thiamin — a substance that helps to protect your nervous system. It also contains iodine which helps to speed up the absorption of iron. Eating it regularly may even prove beneficial in keeping mosquitos away!

Bee Pollen

Pollen is the male reproductive spore of flowering plants. It is collected by female bees in search of nectar, and is formed into pellets by enzymes from the bees' saliva and stored on the hind legs. When bees enter the hive, traps set by the beekeeper brush the pollen pellets off and it is collected and dried for human use.

In writing about this food supplement it should be acknowledged that there are some concerns about exploitation of bees. The main argument seems to be that bees are "enslaved" for production of honey and pollen. Another came in a letter I received after publishing the first edition of *Oakland Organic* in which a reader claimed that the process of collecting pollen with traps results in the occasional loss of a leg by some of the bees. Since I am not a professional beekeeper I cannot verify that claim, though it seems logical. There are 'sustainable' traps that that bees walk across that collect some but not all of their pollen. Other sources on bee pollen claim that bee keepers are able to remove pollen from hives without harming the bees or disturbing their routine.

Bee pollen is about 40% protein, richer than any animal source. It is a natural energizer with carbohydrate and B vitamins. Its amino acids and vitamins make it effective in protecting the skin and treating conditions like psoriasis and eczema. Pollen contains a high quantity of antioxidants, which can have an anti-inflammatory effect on the lungs and prevent the onset of asthma. It is also effective against a wide variety of respiratory diseases and allergies. Pollen contains enzymes that aid digestion and assist your body to obtain nutrients from the food you eat. It supports intestinal flora and yields antibiotic-type properties to boost the immune system. Pollen contains large amounts of *rutin*, an antioxidant that helps strengthen the circulatory system and promotes healthy cholesterol levels. It is even considered to be useful as an aphrodisiac!

With bee pollen a little goes a long way. Just a teaspoonful at mealtime, perhaps sprinkled on yogurt, is all you need to enjoy its healthful effects. Like other foods, the quality of the pollen will reflect the area in which it was gathered. Some pollens are produced in industrial areas and are high in contaminants and low in nutrients. It is best, if possible, to purchase pollen from a known source or 'wild' area that is free of agricultural pollutants such as insecticides. Buy raw bee pollen granules rather than pollen in capsules so that it has not been unnecessarily exposed to light and heat. It should be purchased cool or refrigerated and kept that way when you bring it home.

Propolis

Propolis is a natural antibiotic derived from a sticky coating of leaf buds of trees, used by bees for hive-building material and to encase invaders such as mice or lizards too large to remove from the hive. For thousands of years people have used propolis for its medicinal properties. Greeks used it to treat abscesses. Assyrians put it on wounds and tumors to fight infection and help the healing process. Egyptians used it embalm mummies.

Propolis can be beneficial for throat and mouth irritations including cold sores, stomach ulcers, burns, acne, slow-healing wounds, ear infections, as a treatment for both cancer and diabetes and for cancer prevention. It can be helpful in healing genital herpes and may even protect against radiation. Propolis can be found in lozenge form, tablets, powder and liquid extracts. For topical uses it can be purchased in ointments, creams, lotions and salves and other personal-care products.

Royal Jelly

Royal jelly is a substance secreted from the glands of worker bees to feed their larvae and queens. It has been harvested by humans for centuries for its rejuvenating properties. Queen bees which are fed royal jelly for their entire lives live about 40 times longer than drone or worker bees, largely due to the jelly's nutritional properties.

Royal jelly contains seventeen different amino acids (including all eight essential amino acids, making it a complete protein), most of the B-vitamins, and respectable levels of iron and calcium, essential for blood and bone health. Royal jelly also contains vitamins A, C, and E which are important antioxidants

Research on royal jelly indicates it can be beneficial in multiple ways. For example, the July 1990 edition of the *Journal of Biological Chemistry* reported that a protein found in royal jelly named 'royalisin' provides numerous antibacterial and antimicrobial properties. It aids the skin in collagen production. It can improve insulin resistance and blood pressure because its components may be structurally and functionally related to insulin. Royal jelly fights cancer by suppressing the blood supply to tumors. Since the fatty components of royal jelly exert estrogenic effects, as indicated in a study published in the December 2010 edition of *PLOS One,* the open access peer-reviewed scientific journal, it is possible that royal jelly can treat breast and cervical cancer. It may also help with problems that are related to hormonal imbalance.

Royal jelly is best purchased fresh, since processed forms (such as those found in capsules and extracts) often undergo extensive heating and manufacturing, processes that damage the nutrients and enzymes responsible for providing many of the health benefits. The same considerations for finding bee pollen apply to royal jelly, since where the bees produced it will affect its quality. Bee populations have been rapidly declining, which is thought to be linked to environmental pollution. Support organic, free-range, biodynamic farming and beekeeping practices when possible. Taking about a half-teaspoon a day of royal jelly is enough to enjoy its benefits.

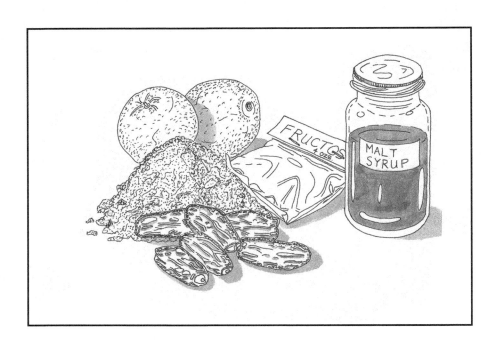

Sugar and Alternative Sweeteners

onald H. Masters, D.D.S. and Howard L. Lewis, writing in *the Journal of the American Society for Preventative Dentistry*, as far back as January 1975, list the following disorders as at least partially caused by too much sugar intake, along with references for their statements:

coronary thrombosis

shortened lifespan

increased dental disease

obesity

high blood pressure

increased triglicerides and cholesterol in blood

dyspepsia

skin diseases and allergies

gouty arthritis

myopia

alcoholism

Excess sugar consumption can put your body on a blood-sugar roller coaster. Since sugar is quickly absorbed, blood glucose rises rapidly, resulting in a surge of energy. But that signals the pancreas to over-secrete insulin to return blood balance to normal. The resulting imbalance pushes the brain and nervous system toward anxiety and depression.

Remember, too that refined sugar is concentrated, unlike the sweet fructose that our ancestors could get from fruit that along with the sugar provides fiber and vitamins and slows down digestion and absorption. Refined sugar contains no vitamins, and foods containing sugars rely on B vitamins, calcium and magnesium for their digestion. Cookies, candies and other foods and drinks containing refined sugars tap into and can deplete your body's stores of these necessary nutrients in their digestive process.

Increasingly, experts believe we can be truly addicted to sugar. As reported in the *UK Telegraph* of Dec. 11, 2014, French scientists in Bordeaux reported that in animal trials, rats chose sugar over cocaine (even when they were addicted to cocaine), and speculated that mammals' sweet receptors are not naturally adapted to the high concentrations of refined sugar available to us in modern times. Research has indicated the same kinds of changes in brain dopamine in animals given intermittent access to sugar as in drug addicts.

Diabetes has become epidemic among Americans: about 10% of Americans have diabetes and 30% are considered pre-diabetic. Prevalence of diabetes among US adults grew by 45% over the past 20 years. Epidemiological research has shown an association between intake of sugar-sweetened beverages and diabetes.

There are more negative findings: a 2013 study found that sugars in the intestine triggered the formation of a hormone called GIP in a process that may in fact affect the cells' susceptibility to cancer formation. And a 2012 paper in the journal *Nature* showed evidence that fructose and glucose in excess can have a toxic effect on the liver similar to the metabolism of ethanol -- the alcohol contained in alcoholic beverages.

When it comes to dental health, there has long been evidence that dietary habits will affect not only individuals, but their offspring. Dr. Weston Price, a practicing dentist who was called by some scientific journals the "Charles Darwin of Nutrition," travelled around the world studying the teeth and gums of indigenous peoples. In his 1939 book, *Nutrition and Physical Degeneration,* he reported that:

> Without exception, he found that 'primitive' people eating diets their ancestors had eaten for thousands of years had perfect teeth structure, wide dental arches, and straight shining teeth free from decay. Gums were also in perfect condition. Without exception, members of these same groups who had abandoned their ancestral diets and were eating Western food, showed narrowed dental arches, crowded teeth, rampant decay and infected gums. (*Better Nutrition*, Oct. 1980)

He concluded that Western methods of commercially preparing and storing foods stripped away vitamins and minerals necessary to prevent these diseases and listed in particular flour, sugar, and modern processed vegetable fat. The alarming idea is that poor diet would not just do damage to existing teeth, but to the facial bone structure of one's offspring, so that the resulting damage to dental health also became a hereditary condition. Of course the positive implication is that by improving diet people can reverse damage to their own teeth as well as promote better outcomes for their children.

Americans consume lots of sugar: an average of 22 teaspoons a day, the equivalent of 355 calories. Yet medical guidelines recommend that women limit themselves to about 6 teaspoons of sugar a day, or 100 calories, and men to about 9 teaspoons a day, or 150 calories. Incidentally, there are 10 teaspoons of sugar in one 12-ounce can of non-diet soda. And sugar may be 'hidden' in our general food supply. You don't have to binge on candy or donuts to get lots of sugar; high fructose corn syrup (HFCS), which is routinely added to make many processed foods more palatable, proves to be a cheap way to add weight and flavor to items such as tomato sauce, fat free dressing, tonic water, marinates, crackers and even bread. Even a cursory review of supermarket labels will show how common HFCS is as an ingredient.

So what alternatives to over-sweetening our lives can we pursue? While it might be nice to believe that honey, molasses or brown sugar are acceptable alternatives since they provide trace minerals and vitamins and in the case of molasses, iron, unfortunately in large amounts they affect the body in the same way as refined sugar. Certainly if you are concerned enough about your health to consider vegetarianism, you'll want to reconsider your relation to candy, donuts, sugary soda and other highly sweetened foods. Just because foods don't contain animal products doesn't mean they are good choices. The sugar habit can be tough to break, but here are suggestions.

If you like soda, try switching to unsweetened sparkling water mixed with fruit juice of your choice. Even better, squeeze fresh orange juice and use that to sweeten beverages. Whenever you can, use sweet foods and their derivatives: date sugar, unsweetened applesauce, bananas, figs and raisins, and even butternut squash. These alternatives are loaded with vitamins, minerals, antioxidants and fiber. The high fiber levels slow carbohydrate absorption, curb appetite and help offset the high fructose content. Pureed cooked apples, bananas or butternut squash can be used in breads, cakes, brownies, ice creams, puddings and smoothies.

Stevia, a nutrient-dense leaf, is a diabetic-friendly substitute available as a powder for baking and general use. Truvia and Xylitol are considered the most natural of artificial sweeteners. Some consider Truvia to be a natural sweetener because it is derived from stevia. Barley malt is a grain-based liquid or powder, high in gluten and antioxidants. Xylitol, often used in sugarless gums and toothpaste, is sold as a white powder with sweetness like that of sucrose. It is naturally found in a variety of fruits and vegetables and plants and is even a by-product of the body's metabolic cycles. Xylitol was first discovered in Finland and made from birchwood trees, and Finnish scientists found that it is non-carcinogenic and does not promote cavities.

The food writer John Calella advised readers of his book *Cooking Naturally* to "desert the desserts." Try substituting for 'junk' foods high in sugar some of the following which in addition to satisfying the sweet tooth provide fiber, pectin, B vitamins, vitamin C, protein and minerals:

dates	prunes	watermelons
figs	grapes	pineapples
raisins	berries	carob

Carob has been used for food for over 5000 years. It offers an alternative to chocolate though it really has an appealing flavor all its own. You can find it in a number of chocolate-like formats: as a powder for baking and mixing into foods, as chips that you can add to cookies, and as a flavoring in candy, baked goods, and hot beverage mixes. Unlike cocoa, carob contains no caffeine or theobromine. Both of these chemicals (which belong to a family of substances called methylxanthines) are stimulants. Both caffeine and theobromine can cause adverse effects such as sleeplessness, jitters, or anxiety if consumed in excessive quantities. Since chocolate is made from cocoa, which is naturally bitter, lots of sugar and fat are added to sweeten chocolate and give it a velvety texture. Because of the natural sweetness of carob much less sweetener is needed to make it into confections. Compared to chocolate, carob is three times richer in calcium, has one third less calories and seventeen times less fat. It also provides minerals and vitamins and is 8% protein. Carob chips sweetened with beet sugar or malted barley can be found in health stores or ordered online. Carob chips and powder are also sold unsweetened, and in vegan (non-dairy) varieties.

There is lots of social and media reinforcement for the idea that we should all indulge in sweet desserts, cinnamon rolls heaped with icing, candy and other 'treats.' Americans are also encouraged to snack frequently on such treats for a quick energy boost. But refined sugar treats should be made the occasional exception to healthier choices. Maybe you don't wish to serve date-sweetened carob cake for your kid's birthday party, but once you move away from highly and unnaturally sweetened foods your craving for them will dissipate to the point where candy and layer cake will seem sickeningly sweet. Apples, grapes, bananas and dates will seem much more appealing and you won't have to worry about undermining your health in the long run. For snacks it is worth looking over offerings in health-oriented markets which typically include dried fruits, trail mixes in many varieties, carob-based treats and natural energy bars. The following chapter offers many suggestions.

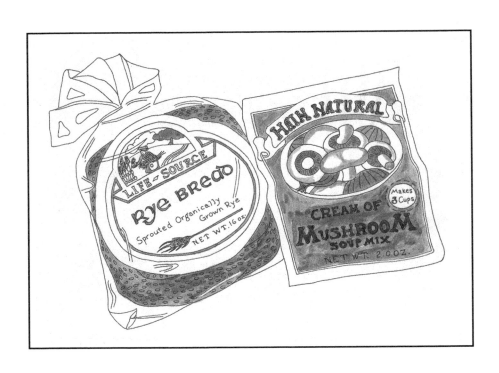

Snacks and Quick Foods

Ideally all of us would stick to several nutritious meals a day and avoid the favorite American pastime of snacking. But realistically, the pace of U. S. jobs and living in general demands occasional quick refreshment. Then again, when people switch to vegetarian diets they are usually eating lighter than they did before. Lunch will no longer be a meatball submarine sandwich that takes a day to digest. So vegetarians may find that five or six smaller meals per day will work better than trying to confine food intake to three larger meals. In either case, there is little excuse to resort to 'junk' foods in desperation for something filling or convenient.

Those who 'brown bag' their lunches have already decided they either must bring food from home or that they prefer their own food to whatever is available at their worksite or from vending machines. So bringing along healthy snacks is a simple matter of including them along with the lunch. In the bigger picture, vegetarians, and any people who take their health seriously will get into the habit of taking along with them some healthful snacks, since fast food and vending machines offer few healthy choices.

Snacks can be simple: a handful of raw almonds or other nuts, trail mix, fresh fruit, carrots, celery or other portable vegetables. Snacks like those will keep all day and are easy to take along. There are other wholesome quick foods you might also try, some more portable than others, but certainly people will want snacks at home too.

RICE CAKES: These have now become a familiar item on the shelves of supermarkets, so they are widely available and make a good light snack, especially when spread with peanut butter, guacamole, hummus or some other topping of your choice. Rice cakes come plain or in blends including rye, corn and sesame seed. One plain rice cake contains between 35 and 70 calories and is 8% protein. It will contain less than 1 gram of total fat, almost none of it saturated fat. So this is a low-calorie, low-fat way to fill yourself up. Rice cakes also provide fiber, iron, zinc and magnesium. You need to choose wisely, however. Big food companies offer rice cakes in versions such as caramel chocolate chip and others that add calories, sugar, fat, excess salt and artificial flavorings. Since rice and other grains are the main ingredients, it is wise to buy brands like Lundberg, make from organic brown rice and flavored naturally with offerings such as toasted sesame, green tea or tamari. That way you will get the most nutrition from this versatile food.

HEALTHY SODAS: While this may seem like a contradiction in terms, there are some sodas that can satisfy the fizz craving without compromising your well-being. You can avoid the artificial colors, preservatives, sugar, and high-fructose corn syrup in typical offerings. For example, Fizzy Lizzy sodas are carbonated water combined with actual fruit juice, with vitamin C added for extra nutrition and no sugar of any kind. Steaz makes no-calorie sodas sweetened with stevia and erythritol, a natural sugar alcohol, and fortified with vitamin B12. Reed's Light Extra Ginger Brew is a "light" variety of ginger ale with 55 calories per bottle, sweetened with honey and stevia. Oogave makes certified-organic sodas that contain half the sugar of conventional sodas. None of their products exceeds 100 calories per bottle and they include flavors such as strawberry-rhubarb and mandarin-key lime. Hansen's natural sodas are perhaps the easiest to find, made with fruit flavors, spices, cane sugar, zero-calorie Splenda® (sucralose) or zero-calorie Truvia™ (made from the stevia plant). You can make your own inexpensive mixes by just adding slices of your favorite fruits and veggies — lemons, oranges, watermelon, cucumber, mint, or limes — to sparkling water for a refreshing and flavorful drink. Or add your favorite fruit juice to seltzer to get a similar mix.

HALVAH: If you are in the mood for candy, this confection offers some redeeming value. Halvah is a traditional sweet found in the Middle East, Greece and Israel, made with a mix of either honey and sesame seeds or sesame seed paste and sugar. So while the sugar does mean some empty calories, the seed content provides significant amounts of several minerals plus some fiber.

Since it's like eating nuts it can satisfy hunger better than just melting a candy bar in your mouth.

ENERGY BARS: Anyone who has been in a health store or even perused the right supermarket aisle has viewed a large selection of energy bars. Here is where reading labels will pay off. Some of these so-called healthy choices are little more than disguised candy bars. Others, similar to halvah, may be sweetened but also contain dried fruit, oats, nuts or seeds which do provide some sustained food and energy value. A Clif bar, for example, uses a combination of organic ingredients, but also weighs in at 230 calories. If you just need a light snack, and are not planning on scaling a rock wall, you might be better off with an apple.

SOY, RICE, COCONUT and ALMOND MILK ICE CREAMS: Even some supermarkets now carry nondairy frozen desserts (other than sorbets and ices) usually made with soy or rice milk, or even coconut or hemp milk. They are arguably healthier than dairy desserts (see this book's Dairy chapter) and allow those who need or want to avoid dairy to indulge in one of life's true pleasures.

SHERBET and SORBET: The main difference between sherbet and sorbet is that sherbet has a small amount of milk fat (1 or 2 percent) and sometimes a bit of egg white or gelatin for texture. Whole fruit sorbet is nondairy and contains puréed fruit among the top three ingredients. This can mean they're healthier, so long as they don't have lots of added sugar. Similarly to nondairy ice creams, if you're vegetarian or allergic to milk or eggs, this can be a great alternative.

CEREALS: Snacking on cereal is a mainstream American habit, but many commercial cereals are bad choices for good nutrition. There is the world of granolas, largely based on rolled oats, but many of those are highly sweetened, usually with a high-calorie content due to the oil used, and are so filling that they are better eaten as a regular meal than as a snack. Better choices are puffed rice, millet, corn, wheat and even kamut. One example is from Arrowhead Mills, which sells puffed cereal in 6-ounce bags which contain whole grain brown rice with no added sugar or salt, and is also fat-free and cholesterol-free with no artificial ingredients. Such 'plain grain' cereals are high in fiber, vitamins and minerals and make for a great snack and will keep well in their bags. They run about 50 calories per cup and can be mixed with nuts and dried fruit to make a light trail mix. Millet is particularly worth trying as it is the most alkaline grain and easy to digest. You can find such puffed cereals in bulk, too, making them an affordable snacking choice.

DRY SOUPS: Dry soup mixes are eminently portable and can be kept for relatively long periods at the workplace or wherever you have a few minutes to add hot water or have access to a microwave. Companies like Dr. McDougall's, Fantastic Foods and Westbrae Natural make vegan soups low in fat and calories, and without the adulterants, preservatives and excess salt of mainstream commercial brands. They come in creative flavors and mixes: Curry with Brown & Wild Rice, Fruited Pilaf, Hot & Sour with Organic Noodles, Miso Soup with Organic Noodles, Pad Thai Noodle, and Black Bean & Lime are just a few of the available varieties.

INSTANT DRINKS: Sometimes you may be more thirsty than hungry, or just want something flavorful to sip that won't give you the jitters.

Postum is one of the original coffee substitutes, around for over 100 years, and when discontinued by the large food manufacturer that originally made it, recreated by Eliza's Quest Foods. The ingredients are roasted wheat bran, wheat, and molasses.

Teeccino is a coffee alternative made with ingredients like barley, chicory, and dandelion, and given sweetness from carob, dates and figs. They have flavors like Vanilla Nut and Maya Chocolate, and can be made with water or almond milk or hemp milk and some stevia to sweeten.

Dandy Blend is another herbal coffee substitute, made with dandelion root. It's gluten-free and tastes good with almond milk and stevia.

Cocoa: You can make cocoa that is healthier than the sugary commercial mixes by using unsweetened vanilla almond milk with a dash of cinnamon and stevia to taste. Add a teaspoon of unsweetened cocoa powder for a chocolatey treat. Unsweetened dark cocoa powder yields many more health benefits than sweetened mix or milk chocolate. Just 1 tablespoon of unsweetened cocoa powder contains 3 to 9 percent of the recommended daily intake of iron, manganese, magnesium and zinc. Also, the flavonoids in dark cocoa function as antioxidants to help prevent systemic inflammation, improve blood flow and help lower blood pressure.

Green tea has less caffeine than coffee and can give you a boost without the jitters. It also contains catechins, powerful antioxidants and disease fighters.

Rooibos tea is full-flavored and mixes well with any kind of milk. It can be a refreshing pick-me-up and may have immune-boosting properties.

Be aware that even decaf coffee has some caffeine; we tested some varieties using caffeine tester strips and all came up with read-outs over 20mg! By comparison, the caffeine content of a cup of regular coffee delivers at least 95mg.

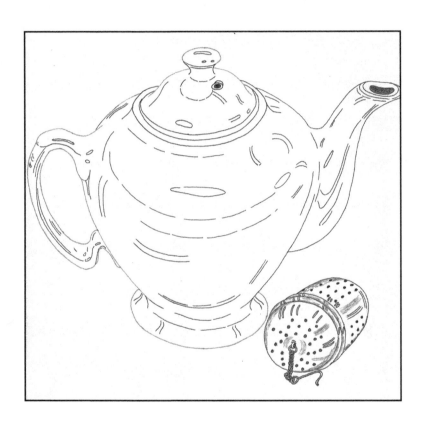

Tea

While many might think of tea as the standard Lipton black tea bag, drinking tea can also be a way to ingest healthful herbs. A cornucopia of herbal, green, white and black tea blends is available in stores in ready-to-use tea bags. These are handy but more expensive that buying tea in loose packs or in bulk, though bulk tea is not as convenient. Even loose-pack premixed teas are more expensive that simply buying your own bulk herbs and mixing them yourself. Many health-oriented stores now offer bulk herbs and loose teas (along with, incidentally, a selection of bulk spices).

While black tea is often consumed as a flavorful alternative to coffee, it delivers half the caffeine. For classic teas, all types are made from the leaves of the plant *Camellia sinensis*, which wilt and oxidize after harvesting. The amount of oxidation determines the different types of teas, from black tea to white tea to green tea. Polyphenols in particular are a group of plant chemicals that are believed to yield health benefits — especially in green tea. The antioxidant benefits of green tea are highly praised by medical researchers. White tea may, in addition, provide even more protection against many types of cancer. Oolong tea falls between green and black tea in that it is partially fermented, providing a fragrant drink with fruity flavor and delivering health benefits similar to green and white teas.

Herbal teas offer many non-caffeinated varieties. Some, like chamomile, are even used to promote relaxation and act as sleep aids. On the other end of the spectrum are stimulating caffeinated teas such as mate leaf from South America and guarana seeds native to the Amazon basin. In between are many herbs and herbal blends that can be used for a variety of medicinal effects. One example is tea made from the Rooibos plant from South Africa, which provides benefits for the immune and circulatory systems, hair and skin, and even anti-aging antioxidants.

To get the most benefit from drinking tea, brewing from bulk is preferable to using tea bags. That's because the leaves used in most bags are "dust and fannings" from broken tea leaves which have lost most of their essential oils and aroma. They release more tannins than whole leaf tea, resulting in bitter brews. And the tea bags themselves keep the tea leaves from expanding to their full flavor and aroma potential.

Some companies offer full-leaf teas packaged in pyramid-shaped bags and tea pouches made of cloth or paper-type materials which allow for fuller infusions that traditional teabags. Metal tea balls are another alternative. There are also tea infusers that fit either a teapot or a cup. One variant is a *gaiwan* to which you add tealeaves and water, brew the tea, then use the special lid to strain the tea as you pour it into a cup.

For best enjoyment and maximum benefit from your tea it is helpful to review how the English make tea. You first need a good teapot, preferably of china or ceramic. Next you need an infuser (a basket or ball to hold the tea leaves in the water) or you can brew the tea loose and use a fine mesh strainer to pour it through when it gets transferred to cups. You can find teapots with built-in infusers which are convenient to use and rinse clean (incidentally, never use soap or detergent to clean your teapot unless you want your tea to taste like soap in the next brewing). Plain water to rinse out the teapot works fine, with perhaps occasional brushing with a bottle-brush or scrubbers if any deposits build up.

If you must substitute a tea ball for a built-in infuser, get one made of stainless steel, not aluminum. Some have two halves which screw together; others work on a hinge; and you can even find single-cup infusers which resemble spoons with hinged lids.

After you decide upon the mixture or variety you'll use for making tea, boil water in a stainless steel kettle, enough to fill the pot. While waiting for the water to boil, fill your pot with hot water from the tap to "warm" it. This is a fine point but makes a big difference in flavor. Fill the infuser-basket or the tea ball with enough herbs for several cups of tea (usually about a teaspoon per cup and "one for the pot" is plenty).

When the water is boiling, pour out the hot water used to warm the pot, and then fill it with boiling water. Lower the tea ball or the infuser into the water (the balls usually have a small hook in the end of a chain to fasten them to the edge of the teapot and make them easier to remove). Put the lid on. Then let the tea steep for at least five minutes, more depending on the strength of tea desired. Stirring once while the tea is brewing will improve flavor and help ensure evenness of brewing.

When the tea has steeped long enough so that you can smell the aroma of the herbs and the water has taken on color, remove the infuser basket of the tea ball. When pouring the tea, if you are pouring two or more cups, fill each cup halfway first, then go back for another round to finish filling the cups. This helps ensure uniformity in the strength of the tea as it's poured. If desired you can add a little honey to enhance the flavor of herb teas. Or you might instead add a little fresh-squeezed orange or lemon juice or some fructose liquid or powder. Some teas are naturally sweet and quite flavorful plain. Another delicious variation is to allow the tea to cool and mix with apple juice (especially delicious with mint teas) or other favorite fruit juices.

Other ways of infusing tea are interesting to try, such as sun and moon infusions. For these methods use a large mason jar or other clear container; put loose teas in proper amount in good water (spring water, or distilled water which tends to draw out the herbs) and set the jar in the sun from morning till night, or in the moonlight from dusk until dawn. You will find in the case of a sun infusion that at the end of the day you will have a delicious tea warmed and infused by the sun's energy; moonlight teas will be more subtle and probably reserved for certain special mixtures (and clear nights!).

Sun infusion works really well with MU tea, a blend of herbs which includes ginseng and other roots and so requires more thorough steeping than leaves. Ingredients for one blend of mu tea include peony root, parsley root, hoelen, cinnamon, licorice, peach kernels, ginger root, ginseng and rhemannia. For blends with hard root herbs and other herbs not in leaf form, adding the mix to water in a saucepan and simmering for ten minutes, then steeping briefly, will bring out the flavor and benefits from the herbs.

Remember that variety is the spice of life, and also a way to avoid dependence on any effects of herbs which are used medicinally. Just as we might warn others to avoid developing a heavy coffee-drinking habit, so it is wise to know and understand the effects of herbs you may brew to drink all day as tea. Herbs are the oldest medicine known to humans, and ought to be treated with due respect and circumspection.

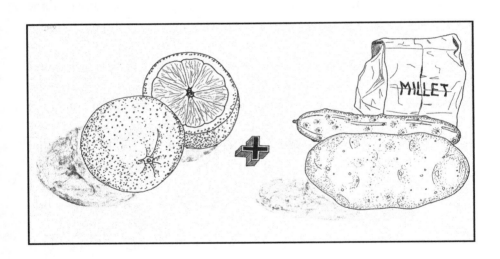

Food Combining

The food combining concept is somewhat controversial. Many health advocates recommend paying attention to which foods you eat together. On the other hand, little formal scientific research has been done to test the theories of food combining.

The basic theory goes as follows: Since protein digestion uses enzymes more acidic than the ones used to digest carbs, when you eat those two types of foods together, the enzymes cancel each other out, so the foods can't be assimilated. Instead, they sit in your digestive system and rot or ferment, building up toxic material in your colon. So according to this theory, you should eat **no proteins and starches at the same meal**.

Another central tenet of food combining is that **fruits and vegetables should not be eaten at the same meal**. That is because fruits are generally acidic food and require different enzymes that will interfere with digestion of starches and with protein digestion which starts with pepsin. In addition, fruits take less time for your digestive system to process compared to heavier foods. However, in fact some foods commonly treated as vegetables are actually fruits, including tomatoes, squashes, peas, beans, and bell peppers.

Lastly, **eat melons alone** is the third food combining precept. The idea is that melons do not digest well with other foods and will therefore cause problems unless consumed alone. There are more complex food-combining schemes than this brief list, but overall the argument leads to the conclusion that the "balanced meals" which present mixes of fruits, vegetables, starches and proteins lead not only to digestive ailments, but to poor assimilation of the nutrients from foods.

Skeptics of food-combining theory argue that the human digestive system will compensate for the variety of foods we may ingest together. It's not just your stomach which does digestive work. Everything you eat, after all, travels through your digestive system. The first stop, the stomach, provides an acid bath to kill bacteria and pathogens and begins to break down proteins. Both carbs and proteins spend time in that acidic environment, although not as long for the carbs. Most digestion and absorption takes place in the small intestine, or duodenum, which produces the different enzymes that digest carbs, proteins, and fats. All of those enzymes are released, no matter what food is in the small intestine. Any undigested food is passed from the small intestine into the large intestine and eliminated from the body as waste. So our digestive system is an amazing and efficient system that we should trust.

According to Michael Picco, M.D., a gastroenterologist with the Mayo Clinic:

> The digestion process takes between 24 and 72 hours, six to eight hours to pass through your stomach and small intestine. Then the food enters your large intestine (colon) for further digestion and absorption of water. Elimination of undigested food residue usually begins after 24 hours. Complete elimination from the body may take several days. (*Mayo Clinic, Digestion: How Long Does it Take?* http://www.mayoclinic. org/digestive-system/expert-answers/faq-20058340)

Different foods will take different lengths of time to move through your digestive system. Melons take the least, from 20 to 30 minutes. Many fruits and vegetables will take approximately 45 minutes. Starchy vegetables such as artichokes, squash, corn and potatoes take about an hour. Concentrated carbs such as rice, cornmeal and oats will take about 90 minutes as will concentrated proteins such as lentils, peas and kidney beans. Soy beans will take 2 hours. Seeds and nuts will take from 2 to 3 hours. Dairy products will take at least two hours, with hard cheeses taking up to 5 hours. Meats such as beef, lamb and pork will also take approximately 5 hours. So in chart form here are approximate digestive times:

Water & Juices: 20-30 minutes
Fruits, Smoothies, Soups: 30-45 minutes

Vegetables: 30-45 minutes
Beans, Grains, Starches: 2-3 hours
Meat, Fish, Poultry: 3 or more hours

Some advice stemming from these differences in digestive times is to eat the foods easiest to digest first in each meal, slowly moving towards the more complex. The analogy is to a highway on which the slower cars will hold up the faster cars behind them, causing a kind of digestive traffic jam.

One other idea is that drinking lots of liquids with a meal will dilute digestive enzymes and so interfere with both salivary and gastric digestion. In particular, too much *cold* water during meals may slow digestion and cause cramping in sensitive individuals. Furthermore, the combined volume of food and water may affect satiety, or the feeling of fullness, since the satiety signal derives in part from pressure sensing. Then again, as water is absorbed quickly we all know that drinking cannot stop hunger by itself. But if you wish to curb your appetite before meals, it may help to drink a glass or two of pure water about 15 to 30 minutes before you eat.

It will depend on the individual as to how much of an impact these food combining guidelines will have on his/her digestion, but they are worth considering if you have problems with gas, bloating or pain after meals. Some health pioneers such as Jethro Kloss (*Back to Eden*) recommend a mono diet: eating one food at a time. While that practice would clearly avoid issues of food combining, for most people it would prove both impractical and too extreme. Even so, the mono diet is probably closest to what primitive humans followed, eating of the food they had just gathered or hunted. Another perspective is that as one's eating progresses to more natural and raw foods, combining foods may prove less problematic. If one simply eats fruits for breakfast, proteins or starch at lunch and salad with either protein or starch for supper, little further thought need be spent upon eating for proper digestion. One thing most people can agree on is that eating too many foods in combination will at least make us drowsy; think of the typical reaction after Thanksgiving dinner. We should not be eating either in quantity or combinations that drive us to seek out digestive remedies such as antacids for reactions like indigestion and heartburn. Certainly overtaxing the digestive system is best avoided if we want to feel energetic and keep our digestive systems in balance. Physicians recommend several smaller meals per day as easier on our systems than a few large meals for these same reasons.

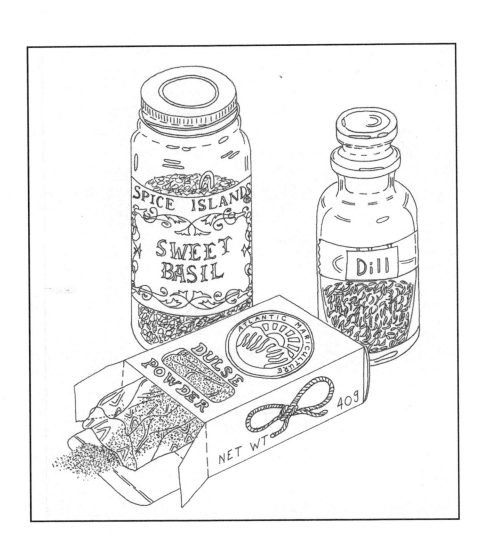

Spices

What happens to my body if I eat too much sodium?

In most people, the kidneys have trouble keeping up with the excess sodium in the bloodstream. As sodium accumulates, the body holds onto water to dilute the sodium. This increases both the amount of fluid surrounding cells and the volume of blood in the bloodstream. Increased blood volume means more work for the heart and more pressure on blood vessels. Over time, the extra work and pressure can stiffen blood vessels, leading to high blood pressure, heart attack, and stroke. It can also lead to heart failure. There is also some evidence that too much salt can damage the heart, aorta, and kidneys without increasing blood pressure, and that it may be bad for bones, too.

--Harvard School of Public Health *(http://www.hsph.harvard. edu/nutritionsource/salt-and-sodium/sodium-health-risks-and-disease)*

As reported by the Rhode Island Dept. of Health, many Americans are eating twice as much salt as is recommended. And much of that excess comes from processed and restaurant foods. Older people should cut down on salt even more. Salt may be "hidden" on labels of ingredients of prepared food under terms like "soda," "sodium" and even the symbol "Na."

Sea salt may be more healthful since it does not contain sugar and other chemicals added to salt in processing, and alternatives such as pink Himalayan salt contain many trace minerals, but the bottom line is these are all basically sodium chloride. Fortunately there are many wonderful herbs and spices to open up worlds of new flavors for foods. Good advice when it comes to salt is to:

- Avoid adding salt to homemade dishes
- Read labels and buy foods with less or no salt
- Eat more fresh food
- Choose unsalted nuts and seeds
- Rinse canned vegetables with water before using (or, of course, choose fresh vegetables instead)
- Limit the amount of salty snacks you eat, like chips and pretzels

Gradually reducing the amount of salt in your food will not be that noticeable. As you wean yourself from salt you will find a great reward in renewed enjoyment of the natural flavors of food—your taste buds will recover from years of assault on their sensitivity and you'll be ready to enjoy more subtle flavorings.

DULSE or sea kelp, available inexpensively in bulk powder or flakes, provides iodine and other minerals and is a good transitional substitute for salt and pepper.

BLACK PEPPER is also a safe spice. While one of its components, safrole, raised some concern due to lab testing decades ago, it remains the most popular spice in the world and you'd have to eat huge amounts over a long period of time to run any risks. It can be an irritant of the GI tract, urinary tract, and prostate, so as with most things, moderation is key. Using a grinder will help you use less to enjoy the full flavor of the peppercorns.

RED PEPPER, a hot spice, provides healthful carotenoids. It can help lower cholesterol and stimulate circulation, and can actually help heal the lining of the stomach.

HERBS come in great variety and can be grown indoors or outdoors, or purchased in bulk and used in many ways with food. Basil, sage, rosemary, marjoram, dill, thyme and the like are well worth keeping on hand.

MINERAL BOUILLON can be used as a liquid seasoning, and as a substitute for its saltier cousin soy sauce. Soy sauce can be found in low sodium versions.

MISO is a favorite seasoning for Asian dishes, make from rice or soybeans and fermented into a paste. (See the "Fermented Foods" chapter). While miso has considerable salt content, it also provides lactobacillus acidophilus, protein and minerals. Also, a small amount provides a lot of flavor.

Cooking with garlic, onions, chili and/or ginger root are additional ways to creatively flavor food and steer away from too much salt. Garlic and onions are praised for their healthful properties, though they can act as irritants to kidneys, the liver and mucous linings of the digestive tract. As with anything else, it is best not to overindulge.

Including lots of organic, fresh, raw foods in your diet will both boost your health and help you to appreciate food's natural flavors. It is also worth trying to avoid automatically spreading foods with salty butter or margarines. You will avoid excess fat calories and may very well better appreciate the foods, such as bread or potatoes, without slathering them in butter, but instead trying some of the seasonings listed above. Olive oil is a more healthful alternative for oil, with true extra-virgin olive oil (EVOO) the best choice. EVOO is extracted from olives using only pressure, a process known as cold pressing. But you may have to be careful to find the real thing, since the U.S. government doesn't regulate the labeling of extra virgin olive oil.

Some tips on buying spices from the U. S. Dept. of Agriculture follow. First of all, spices lose flavor and color during storage and so ideally should be bought in quantities which you will readily use. Health stores will often sell herbs and spices in bulk in any amount from ½ ounce to pounds. After purchase, they keep best in a cool dry place in air-tight containers. You can save small bottles from commercial spices or small plastic containers for storage. Heat hastens flavor loss, and damp can cause caking, color change or infestation. If containers are not tightly sealed after use volatile oils will be lost. Spices will keep with good aroma and flavor for up to six months under favorable conditions. Exceptions are whole spices (nutmeg, cloves, vanilla beans, peppercorn, etc.) which keep flavor indefinitely.

Getting (or growing) fresh herbs and grinding your own whole spices are worth doing for best flavor and full benefits of most of the plants. Try, for example, fresh basil leaves cut up in homemade tomato soup: juice or blend tomatoes and heat with other juiced or chopped vegetables; thicken with arrowroot if desired. Flavor will be much fuller and subtler than when using dry basil leaves as commonly sold. Using a fresh vanilla bean yields a similar surprise in flavor. If dried parsley flakes are all you've ever experienced, buy some fresh parsley which in addition to enhancing flavor and appearance of foods is an herbal blood purifier. Parsley is a healthful and flavorful habit in salads, soups and vegetable dishes.

Ground spices add flavor readily and can be added ten to fifteen minutes before a dish is done cooking, or simply crumbled onto salads and other vegetables. Whole spices can be used for longer-cooking dishes in which simmering extracts full flavor and aroma. Tied in a cheesecloth bag, they are easily removed. Herbs, whole or in leaves, should be crumbled just before use to release flavor. Seeds will be more flavorful if toasted.

You will acquire favorites by experimenting with herbs and spices in your food preparation. Many alternative seasoning mixtures can be sampled from the shelves of your nearest health food store. You may find that you will soon forget salt altogether in favor of the wealth of subtler herbs and spices available, just waiting to be discovered.

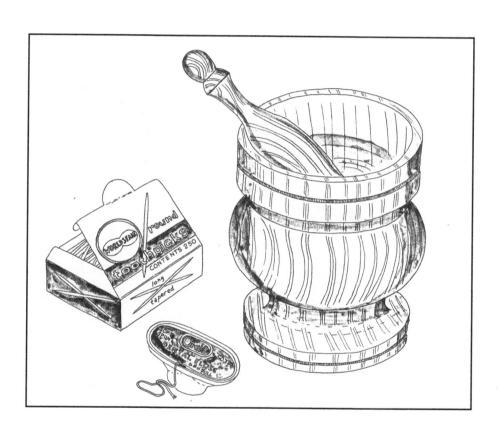

Externals

When discussing health it would be shortsighted to forget about the skin. Your skin is your body's largest and fastest-growing organ. Skin ailments include rashes, dry skin, acne, dermatitis, eczema, psoriasis and skin cancer. It makes sense to take care in protecting this important organ. On average women use more than 200 chemicals on their skin daily and more than 60% of these chemicals get absorbed directly into the bloodstream. Men, too, usually use deodorants, colognes, sun lotions, shaving creams, soaps, shampoos and conditioners.

Many people are unaware that cosmetics are full of dangerous chemicals. More than 500 cosmetic products sold in the U.S. contain ingredients that are banned in Japan, Canada, or Europe. Among those are *petroleum distillates*; *hydroquinone*, a potential carcinogen; *butylated hydroxyanisole* (BHA), linked to endocrine disruption and cancer; *parabens*, suspected endocrine disruptors commonly used in deodorants, and *methyl cellosolve*, a neurotoxin that causes DNA mutation, banned in Canada. These are of course just a small sampling. There are entire websites devoted to listing cosmetics by brand name along with their chemical ingredients so that consumers can be forewarned. It is also worth reflecting that while cosmetic companies may argue that the small amounts of some of these chemicals are negligible, there is no testing for what effects may result from using them in inevitable combinations.

Rather incredibly, but according to their own website, the U. S. Food and Drug Administration does not require that cosmetic manufacturers or marketers test their products for safety! Also if you go to salons, you should be aware that products used by professionals on customers at their establishments are exempt from the requirement to list ingredients on their labels. Overall we have a situation where major cosmetic companies make one batch for Europe and a different batch (with a lot more hazardous chemicals) for the U. S. market. Logic will tell you that either the European Union is being overly cautious, or that U. S consumers are not being protected enough.

Let's track one common ingredient in most shampoos, *sodium lauryl sulfate* (SLS), which generates foam. Actually, foaming is not necessary for shampoos to clean hair, but consumers associate foaming with cleaning. You could, as an alternative, clean your hair with plain baking soda. SLS is considered a "moderate hazard" that has been linked to cancer, neurotoxicity, organ toxicity, skin irritation and endocrine disruption. Yet it is an ingredient in most body washes, soaps, shampoos, and toothpastes. It may also be listed as sodium dodecyl sulfate, sulfuric acid, monododecyl ester, sodium salt, sodium salt sulfuric acid, sodium dodecyl sulfate, aquarex me or aquarex methyl.

SLS is found in a number of industrial cleaning agents such as engine degreaser and industrial strength detergents and can cause irritation of the scalp, gums and skin. Yet it is used as an ingredient in more than 80 products! The *International Journal of Toxicology* recommends concentration levels of no more than 1% in products with prolonged use, but some household soaps have a concentration measurement as high as 30 percent.

You can find shampoos, toothpastes and other personal care products marked "SLS free" and they are not necessarily more expensive than the many that contain this hazardous ingredient. In fact in reference to all cosmetics, another reassurance to look for on the label is the statement, "Not tested on animals." Here again logic tells us that the reason products are tested on animals in the first place is because the manufacturers are well aware that some of the ingredients used may harm humans, so they test them on animals first to see whether they cause rashes or other ill effects, and also to establish a "safe" threshold for the quantity of the chemical that may be included in the formula. If you buy products labeled with "no animal testing," that means there are no ingredients that the manufacturer is concerned about enough to test for harmful effects they may cause to animals.

Toothpaste

Most commercial toothpastes today contain sugar and/or artificial sweeteners…synthetic phosphates of silicas for

abrasion...synthetic glycerin from petroleum, preservatives,
a synthetic chemical for product smoothness...

--Tom's of Maine pamphlet

While it may not matter a great deal what you use for brushing so far as abrasive qualities of the paste or powder, you'll want to avoid the same colorings, chemical additives and undesirable ingredients that are often used in cosmetic formulas. "You will brush your teeth 1,000 times per year or more, and each time you do, you will ingest some toothpaste. If you think that is not a problem, think again," says Dr. Harold Katz of NewsUSA. As with cleaning your hair, you can brush your teeth effectively with plain baking soda, though most people prefer something in a tube with better flavor.

Look for toothpaste with natural ingredients like Aloe Juice and Tea Tree Oil. Xylitol is an excellent cavity fighting sweetener... And avoid toothpastes with added colors -- they serve no purpose and can actually decrease the whiteness of your teeth over time.

-- Dr. Harold Katz, NewsUSA *(http://www.newsusa.com/ articles/article/toothpaste-ingredients-dentists-say-to-avoid.aspx)*

Another alternative is to make you OWN toothpaste. Here are two recipes from *The Herbalist* by Joseph Meyer: (published by Indiana Botanic Gardens, 1934)

I.
Mix a small amount of powdered sage with one ounce of myrrh, grinding to a fine powder.

Mix carefully : 1 pound powdered arrowroot
3 ounces powdered orris root
20 drops oil of lemon
10 drops oil of cloves
12 drops oil of bergamot
Rub oils with powders until well-mixed, then brush!

II.

Mix ingredients to consistency desired:

> ½ ounce powdered chalk
> 3 ounces powdered orris root
> 4 teaspoons tincture of vanilla
> 15 drops oil of rose geranium
> Honey, enough for desired consistency

Keep in a small airtight container.

General oral health also means avoiding too many sugary foods which produce acids that can damage your teeth. Toffee and other sticky candies, sugary chewing gum, sugary drinks including sodas and sweetened sports drinks, are obviously a bad idea. So too are sticky dried fruits unless you make sure to rinse your mouth well afterward. Some breakfast cereals, and breads, especially those made with bleached white flour which has little nutritional value in the first place, can also be classified as acidic. Drinking and rinsing with water or chewing sugarless gum after eating something acidic can help wash away acid, or stimulate saliva to neutralize it.

It is also instructive to reflect that "if your diet consists largely of nutritionally poor foods, your oral health is bound to suffer. That's because **your immune system needs a balance of minerals and vitamins in order to fight infection.** Some research shows that if you aren't eating a nutritious diet, you're more vulnerable to tooth decay and gum disease" (Lisa Bendall, *Five Foods Your Dentist Wants You to Avoid*, besthealthmag.ca). Furthermore, problems with teeth and gums can result from atrophy; living on a diet of soft and prepared foods means that the mouth and jaw are not properly exercised. So here are yet more reasons to drop the junk food and snack on some raw carrots!

See more information about the astonishing findings of the dentist Dr. Weston Price in the "Sugar and Alternative Sweeteners" chapter.

Baths

> People have been using mineral springs and various kinds of
> mineral water baths for ages, long before civilization…The

available research work, corroborated by our own experience, suggests that inorganic minerals present in seawater and mineral waters have a definite cumulative effect on many disorders by stimulating the body's own defensive and healing forces.

--Dr. Paavo Airola, *Are You Confused?*
Phoenix: Health Plus, 1987

If you happen to live within visiting distance of natural hot springs you can enjoy the benefits of natural mineral waters. Otherwise you may not be able to afford regular visits to a famous healing spa. But you can purchase packets of salts similar to those found in hot mineral springs, typically Epsom salt and natural sea salt. When dissolved in hot water, such bath salts can help relieve aches and pains, relax tired muscles and refresh the body. If you add essential oils and/or dried herbs you can also enjoy the soothing effects of aromatherapy.

If you have no bathtub, you can turn your shower into a version of Scandinavian sauna therapy. Dr. Paavo Airola makes this recommendation in *Swedish Beauty Secrets* (Health Plus Publishers, June 1972):

There is unanimous agreement among the foremost experts on beauty and health that constant temperature changes are invigorating and stimulating on the biochemical activity of the skin. Fresh, cool air and outdoor activities stimulate blood circulation and bring more blood to the outer layers of the skin.

Take once or twice a day an alternative warm and cold shower, preferably in connection with your daily exercises. Start with warm water and make three or four changes from warm to cold during each shower. Specifically, expose your face to the cold and warm changes. Always finish with cold water and rub yourself dry with a coarse towel or bristle brush.

Skin Creams

Moisturizing lotions can help prevent dry skin for both men and women. *Aloe vera*, derived from a succulent plant, can be helpful for a variety of skin disorders. In addition to moisturizing it may be helpful for first- and second-degree burns. Aloe is safe in small doses and is even edible. *Aloe vera* gel is used commercially as an ingredient in yogurts, beverages, and some desserts. It is also comparatively inexpensive. Commercial moisturizing lotions are available using aloe vera as a primary ingredient.

Another skin preparation worth knowing about is Tiger Balm. This preparation from Singapore, Malaysia was originally developed during the 1870s in Rangoon, Burma, by the son of a Hakka herbalist in China. The balm promises relief from minor muscle aches and pains and is made of various oils (clove, cassia, peppermint, cajaput) in a petroleum jelly/paraffin base with camphor and menthol. It feels soothing when applied to the forehead and allowed to slowly evaporate, providing a delicious cooling sensation, and can be a wonderful alternative to aspirin. Apply to the chest and upper lip for respiratory congestion.

If you are concerned about petroleum jelly or simply wish to make a version of Tiger Balm at home, try the following recipe:

> Mix together and heat 1/2 ounce of beeswax and approximately 2 ounces of coconut or extra-virgin olive oil in a double boiler, or place a small saucepan inside another to make your own double boiler. Place water to heat in the bottom pot or pan, and place a smaller saucepan for mixed ingredients inside that one. Heat this mixture over low heat, stirring constantly until it's melted. Then remove from heat.

> Add approximately 10 drops each of peppermint and eucalyptus oils and about five drops of clove oil. Mix and stir these essential oils into the beeswax and olive oil mixture thoroughly. Allow the heated mixture to cool for several minutes.

Add fresh herbs to the mixture if you desire. Herbs such as garden sage, wintergreen, black haw and willow are effective in the treatment of aching muscles and joints, says Project Aware. To prepare the herbs for inclusion in the Tiger Balm recipe, boil roughly 1 tablespoon herbs (or more if you wish) in a pint of water. Boil for several minutes until liquid is reduced by half.

Strain the herbs from the water infusion, and add desired amount of infused herbal water into the mixture of beeswax and olive oil. Heat this mixture until the water has evaporated. Allow the mixture to cool for five minutes.

Pour the oil mixture into a clean, medium-size glass or metal container. Let stand until completely cooled.

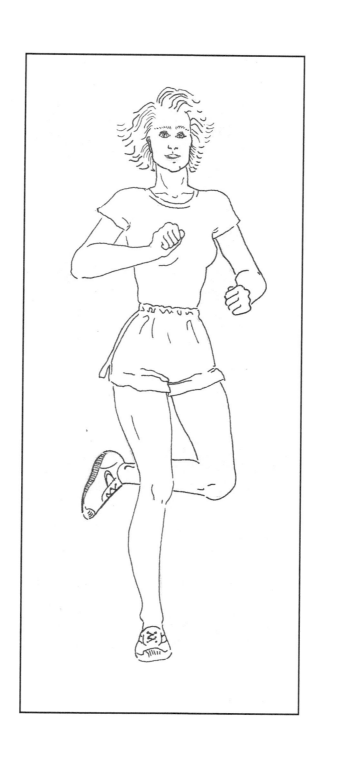

Exercise and Extras

Regular aerobic exercise can bring remarkable changes not just to your body, your metabolism, and your heart, but also to your spirits, reports the February 2011 issue of Harvard Men's Health Watch. Aerobic exercise is the key for your head, just as it is for your heart. It has a unique capacity to exhilarate and relax, to provide stimulation and calm, to counter depression and dissipate stress. Endurance athletes commonly experience the restorative power of exercise, and this has been verified in clinical trials that have used exercise to treat anxiety and depression.

--Harvard Health Publications, *Benefits of Exercise (http:// www.health.harvard.edu/press_releases/benefits-of-exercise)*

Eating the best organic vegetarian diet conceivable may not, in and of itself, lead to optimum health, for food is but one part of a healthy approach to life. Sunshine, clean air and water, exercise, proper rest and relaxation, tranquil thoughts and positive attitudes, yoga or other physical and spiritual disciplines and even other supportive people are also sources of 'nutrition' equally important as food and food supplements.

It would be hard to find any physician or health professional who does not recommend exercise at least a few times a week. According to the Mayo Clinic (*Exercise, 7 Benefits of Regular Physical Activity*) exercise provides many benefits:

Exercise helps prevent excess weight gain or helps maintain weight loss.

It helps prevent or manage a wide range of health problems and concerns, including stroke, metabolic syndrome, type 2 diabetes, depression, certain types of cancer, arthritis and falls.

It improves mood--you may feel better about your appearance and yourself when you exercise regularly, which can boost your confidence and improve your self-esteem.

It boosts energy--exercise and physical activity deliver oxygen and nutrients to your tissues and help your cardiovascular system work more efficiently. It also supplies the brain with an increased amount of oxygen and essential nutrients.

It strengthens and builds bones.

It promotes better sleep.

Regular physical activity can lead to enhanced arousal for women. And men who exercise regularly are less likely to have problems with erectile dysfunction than are men who don't exercise.

It can be fun; it gives you a chance to unwind, enjoy the outdoors or simply engage in activities that make you happy. Physical activity can also help you connect with family or friends in a fun social setting.

Each person will have individual preference for the type of exercise. It might be organized sports played on teams, or sports that can also be individual such as jogging or swimming. Even housework and walking briskly count as moderate exercise. The bottom line is a minimum of 30 minutes at moderate intensity for at least four days of the week, in any cumulative combination. That means that 3 or 4 shorter sessions of 10 or 15 minutes of activity will give the same benefits as a sustained one-hour workout, so there is plenty of choice for how we go about exercising, and as a corollary it is hard to argue that most people can't find 2 hours per week for engaging in activities that yield so many benefits.

Exercise, like most activities we repeat frequently, becomes a habit. If you exercise regularly you get used to the feeling of being in better shape, the feeling of being less stressed, and the enjoyment of the endomorphin effect, noted in this description from WebMD:

> When you exercise, your body releases chemicals called endorphins. These endorphins interact with the receptors in your brain that reduce your perception of pain.
>
> Endorphins also trigger a positive feeling in the body, similar to that of morphine. For example, the feeling that follows a run or workout is often described as "euphoric." *(http://www. webmd.com/depression/guide/exercise-depression)*

Once you get the habit of exercising, you feel worse if you DON'T exercise, which motivates you to continue. And there is no age limit to exercise, nor is there some arbitrary age at which you must give up your favorite activities so long as you are in condition to do them. Though I am at typical "retirement" age I still enjoy jogging, playing soccer, roller blading, swimming, and hiking. Fauja Singh, a vegetarian, born in 1911, completed several marathons though he is over 100 years old! He holds the world record for age 90+, set at the 26-mile Toronto Waterfront Marathon in 2013.

At the intersection of exercise and nutrition, a vegetarian diet may be ideally suited to good performance. In an article published in *Runners World* (May 1978) Dr. Julian Whitaker referred to studies supporting these points:

> High fat foods such as eggs, meats, cheese and dairy products markedly reduce the oxygen supply to the tissues...Fat-induced oxygen deprivation presents serious health problems. Lower fat foods such as grains, fruits and vegetables are oxygen foods, or running foods.
>
> Complex carbohydrate foods are ideal for the runner. Unlike fats, they are completely digested and do not cause clumping

of the red blood cells. As an energy food they are far superior to proteins which are not utilized to any great extent in endurance activities.

Dairy products may not be the best choice for marathon running. About 75 percent of the world's population is genetically unable to properly digest milk and other dairy products — the problem called lactose intolerance. And as we age the enzyme needed to help digest milk sugar decreases in the stomach lining. For these reasons some runners and sports medicine experts warn of nausea, diarrhea or vomiting after a run linked to consuming dairy products.

Note that such recommendations come from people focused not on vegetarianism or even health per se, but on athletic accomplishment, or optimal performance from the healthy body. Yet they confirm similar findings by health researchers referred to in other chapters of this book, such as "Dairy Products" and "Alternative Protein."

The category of good nutrition referred to as "tranquil thoughts and positive attitudes" sounds less concrete and easy to grasp as plain old "exercise," yet the two are closely related. Remember, the body and mind are connected. Your brain is also a physical organ requiring a steady blood supply. At the same time, we are familiar with psychosomatic effects. Headaches typically begin with some mental trigger or in response to stress, but wind up manifesting with physical pain. There is also the well-known placebo effect, routinely used to test new drugs. Many people given a sugar pill, who believe they are receiving medical attention, will experience an improvement in their condition, even though they in fact did not receive medication. An impressive if gruesome example of mind over matter was displayed during protests by Buddhist monks in South Vietnam in 1963. Quang Duc immolated himself in a Saigon intersection, and as reporter David Halberstam wrote, "As he burned he never moved a muscle, never uttered a sound, his outward composure in sharp contrast to the wailing people around him" (Halberstam, David (1965), *The Making of a Quagmire*, New York: Random House). Imagine training your mind to turn off physical pain so completely that you could sit calmly in the lotus posture while you literally burned to death. While it may not have been his primary purpose, Quang Duc and others who repeated his protest clearly demonstrated the power of mind over matter.

Yoga has become increasingly popular in the West since the first publication of this book, and for good reason. Yoga is system that involves physical postures, breathing exercises and meditation, all three of which are interwoven and essential to pursuing yogic culture. Yoga therefore combines both the physical (stretches, breathing and postures) and the mental (meditation and relaxation techniques) which together lead to physical improvement and tranquil thoughts and positive attitudes. There are many books and classes with which to get introduced to the practice of yoga. Two classics are *Light on Yoga* by B. K. S. Iyengar and *The Complete Illustrated Book of Yoga* by Swami Vishnudevananda. I started yoga practice rather skeptically but soon found it so rewarding in terms of feeling physically better, reducing stress and facing life more calmly that I have kept it up ever since. Even a few stretches and some brief breathing and meditation each day will bring big rewards. At the same time yoga practice can become quite advanced, yielding even more benefits.

If yoga seems inaccessible to you at present, consider some positive philosophies toward life to counteract the easier-to-find cynical and negative ones. You can seek out and use such wisdom as helpful affirmations. Here is an example from Neal Cassady as recorded by Jack Kerouac, which can be found in the book *Scenes Along the Road* by Ann Charters. A photograph of Cassady at the wheel speaking to a woman carries the subtitle, "Neil in heaven—an old car and a girl":

> Now you just dig them in front. They have worries, they're counting the miles, they're thinking about where to sleep tonight, how much money for gas, the weather, how they'll get there—and all the time they'll get there anyway, you see. But they need to worry and betray time with urgencies false and otherwise, purely anxious and whiny, their souls really won't be at peace unless they can latch on to an established and proven worry and having once found it they assume facial expressions to fit and go with it, which is, you see, unhappiness, and all the time it all flies by them and they know it and that too worries them no end. (City Lights Books, June 1985)

One last consideration about mental health concerns that of others. There are people who will add to your life, and others who may prove to be a drain on your spirits and energy. Along with the serenity attainable through yoga practice comes the desire to avoid stressful situations, to keep the peace and balance with which you attempt to begin and end each day. You may need to reappraise your relationships with people who figure prominently in your life: fellow employees, friends, bosses, significant others. If you realize that certain persons exert a negative drain on your energy and well-being, you may need to reevaluate their role in your life, at least until such time as they may learn to communicate from a more balanced attitude. If you must change jobs, move, find different friends or lovers, so be it. If you do not follow your instincts, but let others stunt your psychic growth, then both of you will suffer. Perhaps this is the wisdom behind the old proverb that people can be judged by the company they keep.

Remember that the central aim of good health will be served by trying to live in a calm manner. You can practice this in other ways besides yoga. If you're stuck in a traffic jam, why grit your teeth and curse all the other cars and drivers? Better to relax, listen to the radio or think constructive thoughts, since essentially you are powerless to change your immediate situation. By attending to this principle you will find other ways to spare yourself needless stress and frustration.

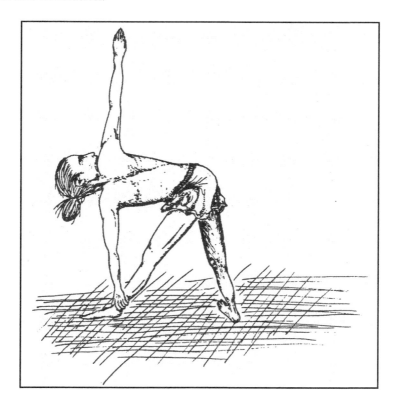

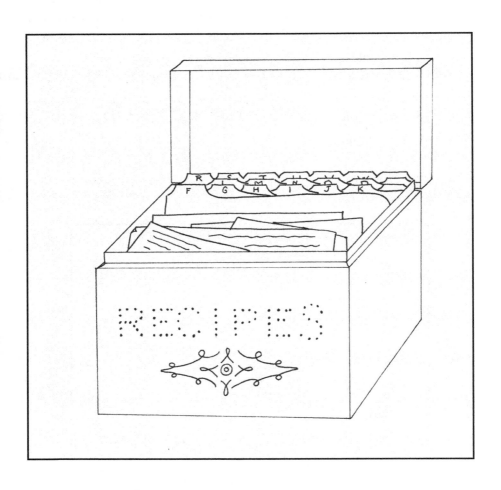

Recipes

There are many books with good recipes for vegetarians and vegans. As just a few examples, the *Forks Over Knives* cookbook offers "over 300 recipes for plant-based eating throughout the year." There is even a cookbook for kids: *Plant-Powered Families.* Some derive recipes from traditional cultures, such as *Vegan Richa's Indian Kitchen* or *Cloe's Vegan Italian Kitchen.* And there are sub-specialties for raw vegan baking such as *Rawsome Vegan Baking* and *Artisan Vegan Cheese.* There are guides for weight loss such as *Appetite for Reduction: 125 Fast and Filling Low-Fat Vegan Recipes.* And there are vegan websites that offer free recipes: Allrecipes.com offers 1370 of them, and PETA invites browsers to "browse hundreds of free recipes."

With all these choices, there is no need for this book to list too many, but a few follow that include some originals. Then too, as Jethro Kloss noted in his classic *Back to Eden,* once principles of healthful eating are realized there is little need for recipes—the simpler the fare the better. Nevertheless reading recipes can stimulate one to try unfamiliar foods and increase variety in the diet.

SAVORY DISHES

DENIS MEXICAN

Steam either organic corn or whole wheat tortillas.

Mixing cold-pressed oil and water equally, stir-fry a medium onion until soft.

Drain one can of cooked soybeans, saving the liquid (rich in lecithin) for soups or drinking. Or use one to two cups of fresh-cooked soybeans; add to onion and crush with fork.

Add several Ts enchilada sauce (or fresh-blended sauce with hot spices) and a diced fresh tomato and heat together thoroughly. Parsley or basil make fine garnishes.

Spoon mixture onto steamed tortilla, add avocado and/or lettuce and roll up, with perhaps extra enchilada sauce on top.

YEAST CAKES

Mix together:
    1 cup yeast flakes
    ½ cup wheat germ
    several grated or ground carrots
    2 – 3 T oil or salad dressing
    1 cup water
    favorite spices

Add water last and stir to make smooth. Fry in mixture of water and oil until browned on both sides. Serve with sprouts and salad.

This recipe may also be made slightly thinner (add more water) and used for eggless omelets; flip when edges get crisp, fill with onion, green pepper, sprouts, spinach, mushrooms, etc., then fold in half and brown on both sides.

YEAST CAKE II

½ cup wheat germ
½ cup whole wheat flour
1T broth powder
1 tsp dulse powder
Sesame seeds
1T miso
3T tomato paste or medium fresh tomato, crushed

Mix these with 1 cup water until smooth; cook as for Yeast Cakes above.

BREAD SPREAD

Blend mung and other sprouts and add broth powder or vegetable seasoning, nutritional yeast, soy sauce or Bragg liquid seasoning, and paprika. Use an as all-purpose dressing and spread. If you use sprouted peas or soybeans, you may wish to cook them slightly.

PAM'S PEPPERS

4 green peppers
2 and 1/2 cups cooked brown rice
1 onion
1 clove garlic
1T sunflower seeds, shelled
1T sesame seeds
½ cup raw nuts
½ cup raisins or currants
1/3 cup cranberry or grape juice
3T soy sauce

Sauté onion & garlic with a little oil in large pan until softened (mixing a little water with the oil will give the best result). Add seeds, nuts and raisins and fruit juice and soy sauce. Mix thoroughly, cover pan and simmer for 15 minutes.

Cut peppers ½ inch from top and save tops for later. Remove pith and stand peppers next to each other in oiled loaf pan. Preheat oven to 350 degrees.

When roasted nutty mixture is done, toss in a bowl with rice. Divide the mixture among the four peppers and pack firmly. Replace tops on the peppers and bake for 20 – 30 minutes.

SWEET FOODS

BAKED APPLES (with miso)

Prepare sesame-raisin miso:
    2T sesame butter or ground seeds

¼ cup raisins
1T miso
1T soy margarine or oil
2T honey, fructose or molasses
2T water
½ tsp cinnamon

Mix above ingredients, pack into cored apples (do not cut through apples all the way—leave bottoms in). Wrap apples in foil, place on cookie sheet and bake at 350 degrees for about 30 minutes. Serve hot or cold.

PRUNE-NUT BUTTER BALLS

Mix together in saucepan:
3 cups chopped pitted prunes
2/3 cup water
1/3 cup peanut or almond butter
Cook together for 10 minutes, stirring until thick. Stir in:
2/3 cup chopped walnuts (or cashews)
2/3 cup granola
½ cup flaked coconut

Allow to cool, then shape into golf ball-size pieces, roll in more flaked coconut and refrigerate.

FRUIT SPREAD

1cup dried raisins
1 cup dried pears
1 cup dried apples
2 cups apple juice (or water)
2T vegetable oil
1 cup nuts, finely chopped

Combine fruits and juice in a saucepan and simmer until all are soft. Blend. Mix in oil and favorite spice. Refrigerate. (Christiane Munkholm Levy, Talking Food Co.)

CLOVERDALE FRUIT CAKE
(same credit as for above recipe)

3T dried yeast	1 tsp salt
½ cup lukewarm apple juice	1 cup prunes, pitted & chopped
½ cup honey	1 cup dried apricots, pitted & chopped
½ cup oil	1 cup dates, chopped
3 eggs (substitute applesauce if you do not wish to use eggs)	
1 cup cold apple juice	½ tsp ground anise seed
1 ½ cups whole wheat flour	½ tsp grated lemon rind
1 ½ cups rye flour	½ cup sesame seeds
	½ cup sunflower seeds

In large bowl, soften yeast in warm juice. In small bowl, blend honey and oil, then add eggs one at a time. Combine with softened yeast and cold cider in large bowl. Stir in flours and salt. Mix fruits and seeds and blend into batter. Turn into oiled 12" x 8" cake pan and let set in a warm place until slightly risen. Bake one hour at 350 degrees.

FRUITED ASPIC

¼ oz agar (1 bar kanten or 2½ T flakes or ½oz Irish moss without kelp)
4 cups water (or mix water with up to 2 cups apple, grape, or orange juice)
Juice of ½ lemon
1 – 4 T honey to taste
1 cup fresh fruit (or rehydrated)
½ cup chopped nuts
pinch of kelp (in place of salt)

In six-cup saucepan soften agar in 2 cups water, then cook quickly over medium heat until dissolved. Reduce to simmer, stir in honey with remaining 2 cups water or juice. Remove from heat and blend in lemon juice and kelp (if desired). Rinse 6-cup mold or serving dish in cool water, arrange fruit on bottom and sides. Pour slightly cooled agar mixture over the fruit and leave until partially set, then add layer of chopped nuts and allow to set thoroughly.

PARADISE CITRUS PUDDING

1 cup carrot juice
½ unripe papayas

Blend. In minutes enzyme reaction produces a delicious pudding. Will thicken more when cooled.

(from *Survival into the 21ˢᵗ Century* by V. Kulvinskas, p. 253)

TOFU CHEESECAKE

3 cups tofu
1/3 cup fresh lemon juice
¼ cup oil plus ¼ cup soy margarine, melted & cooled
½ cup honey
½ tsp salt
1 tsp vanilla
¼ cup soymilk or water, if necessary

Combine ingredients in a blender in order given, adding liquid at the end only if needed to blend tofu. Mixture should be fairly thick, of creamy consistency. Pour into crumb crust (see below) and bake approximately ½ hour at 350 degrees or until tofu is set in the middle (a knife blade inserted should come out clean). Topping can be fresh strawberries or cherries or blended fruits.

CHEESECAKE CRUST

2 cups unbleached or whole wheat pastry flour
½ cup honey
¼ tsp salt
dash cinnamon
2T oil

½ cup softened soy margarine
2T water

Mix dry ingredients. Work in oil and margarine with fingers. Work in water. Pat on bottom and halfway up side of pan. Partially bake for 10 minutes at 350 degrees. Fill with cheesecake mix and bake as above. Be careful—this crust burns easily.

An alternative recipe uses GRAHAM CRACKERS, which can be found in wholesome whole wheat versions:

1½ cups graham cracker crumbs – they can be crumbled in a blender
1/3 cup melted butter
1/3 cup honey or sugar

Mix all ingredients together and press into the bottom of springform or pie pan. Bake at 350 degrees for 8 – 10 minutes. Cool and fill with cheesecake mix and bake as above.

INSTANT CRUST

Use a package of about one dozen health cookies, preferably a soft, crumbly variety. Simply line your pan, then fill with the cheesecake mixture with no prebaking.

CLAUDE'S CAKE (macrobiotic)

1 cup whole wheat flour
½ cup buckwheat flour
½ cup chestnut flour
½ cup unbleached flour
½ cup soy flour
½ tsp sea salt
2T oil
1T tahini
apple juice and water, mixed ½ & ½
1 tsp self-rising yeast

1 egg
6T raisins
pinch cinnamon
grated orange peel

Mix flours, add salt and work oil and tahini into the mix. Let stand 20 minutes. Mix 1 tsp yeast with ¼ cup water; work into mix. Mix in egg and orange peel. Add raisins. Mix all ingredients with apple juice & water until wet and elastic. Flour the dough and place in greased pan. *Let stand overnight.* Bake at 375 degrees for and 1½ hours.

(from *Zen Macrobiotic Cooking* by Michael Abehsara)

MACROBIOTIC PUDDING
(using Claude's Cake recipe)

Soak one pound of organic dried fruit (peaches, pears, apples) overnight to soften. Put in blender with enough honey to sweeten taste plus some of your favorite sweet spices, and reduce to pudding consistency. Crumble Claude's Cake into a bowl and fold in fruit paste to achieve a firm, smooth pudding. Garnish and serve. For festive occasions, a little sherry or rum will enhance the flavor.

LICIA'S NEW AGE HEALTH PUDDING

2 cups water
1 cup apple juice
4T arrowroot or 6T agar-agar
1½ tsp vanilla
6 – 8 T powdered carob
½ cup honey
¼ cup molasses or malt syrup
¼ cup raisins

Heat water and apple juice in a saucepan. Dissolve arrowroot and agar-agar in enough cool water to make a smooth paste. Add all ingredients to saucepan, heat until mixture is thick and bubbling, stirring frequently, and cook for several minutes. Pour into serving dishes or molds and chill.

COLD CAROB PUDDING

3 – 4 T roasted carob powder
1T bee pollen
1T whey powder
1T nutritional yeast
1T fructose to sweeten (optional)
Bran, wheat germ, orange juice

Mix dry ingredients in bowl, using wheat germ and/or bran as desired. Add orange juice or water gradually, moistening dry mix until desired thickness is achieved. This pudding will thicken when refrigerated.

BAKED DISHES

CARROT PULP CAKE

2½ cups carrot pulp (from juicing)
¾ cup whole wheat flour
½ cup molasses
½ cup honey
1 tsp baking soda or powder
½ cup raisins
½ cup chopped nuts
2 tsp cinnamon
1 tsp cloves/allspice

Bake at 350 degrees for one hour, or until knife comes out clean and edges of cake are a bit browned. Frost with Apricot Icing (below):

1½ cups dried apricots, soaked & softened
1/3 cup honey (to taste)
2 – 3T dry milk powder or soyamel (powdered soy milk) or Tiger's milk
soaking water to thin

Blend ingredients to make a smooth, thick paste. Spread on cooled cake.

WHEAT GERM STICKS

2 cups whole wheat flour
1 cup wheat germ
¼ cup sesame seeds (unhulled)
½ cup coconut
3 T honey
1 tsp salt
½ cup oil
1 cup yogurt or blended tofu (or water or broth)

Mix ingredients and roll out ½ inch thick. Cut sticks ½" x 4" long. Bake at 350 degrees on oiled cookie sheet for 30 minutes, until slightly brown.

SPROUTED WHEAT STICKS

Soak wheatberries overnight (8 hours)

Using large jars with cheesecloth or screen closing tops, allow berries to sprout for 24 hours or until shoots appear; rinse and drain 2 or 3 times per day.

Blend sprouted wheatberries with enough soak liquid to broth to make a thick paste. Add broth powder or spices if desired.

Bake at 350 degrees for about ½ hour or until crisp (on foil or oiled baking sheet) OR sun-dry until crisp (about 2 hours) turning over once.

Serve plain or with miso.

STEAMED DISHES

CAROB TEA BREAD

¾ cup carob powder
1½ cups mashed sweet potatoes or pumpkin or squash
1 cup rolled oats
3 cups rye flour
1¾ cups honey (or less, to taste)
1 cup cornmeal

1 cup cooked brown rice

2½ cups soy milk

1 tsp salt (sea) or kelp

1½ cup raisins

Mix ingredients and fill a large mold, empty can or oven-proof bowl, then cover with tin foil. Steam on a rack in a covered pot for two and a half hours if using the bowl or mold, or two hours for the can. Or steam in a pressure cooker in at least 5 cups of water for 30 minutes or more. Store fully cooled loaves in refrigerator for a few days to 'ripen' for best results. Slices can be toasted or resteamed before serving.

SOYSAGE (steamed main dish)

4 cups pulp from making soymilk, or cooked cracked soybeans

2 cups whole wheat flour

1 cup wheat germ

¾ cup oil

1 cup nutritional yeast flakes

1½ cups fennel seed

1 tsp kelp

¼ cup soy sauce

3 tsp oregano

½ tsp cayenne

2 T garlic powder or 2 cloves crushed fresh garlic

2 tsp mustard or 1 tsp dry mustard

2 tsp allspice

Mix all ingredients and prepare for steaming as above. Steam in large pot of water for 1½ hours, or pressure cook for 30 minutes. Cool and slice for frying or resteam to serve. Closest taste to sausage this side of meat, thoroughly nutritious.

(from *Farm Vegetarian Cookbook*, p. 146)

FROZEN FOODS

FRUIT SHERBETS
(adopted from *Cooking Naturally* by John Callela)

With the aid of a Champion or Acme juicer, the following ingredients and similar variations can be turned into wonderful frozen confections:

ORANGE/PINEAPPLE

3 cups mixed orange and pineapple juice
½ pineapple, diced
3 oranges, diced
2T lecithin granules
2T soyamel (powdered soymilk) or protein powder
1 tsp vanilla

BANANA-DATE-FIG

3 cups fig juice
2 bananas
6 dates
2T soyamel
1 tsp carob powder

1. Combine juices with other ingredients in blender.
2. Pour blended mixture into freezing trays and freeze solid.
3. Cut frozen mix into thin strips which will fit into the throat of your juicer.
4. Assemble juicer for homogenizing and process frozen strips.

Serve immediately, or store in paper or plastic containers in freezer for later.

SOY ICE BEAN

Follow basic recipe instructions above, using 3 cups of freshly made soy milk combined with other desired sweeteners, carob powder, fruits and juices. Including a few tablespoons of agar-agar will ensure jelling and a few tablespoons of vegetable oil will help smoothness.

BEVERAGES

SAIGE & DARCY'S SMOOTHIE

Fill your blender about 1/3 full with frozen organic fruits (sold in bags in markets)
Add enough soy or rice milk to cover the fruit
Add an equal amount of fruit juice of your choice
Add one scoop of vegan protein powder (no whey)
Add a banana and other fresh fruit
Optional: one or tablespoons peanut or almond butter
You can also add yogurt for a thicker shake
For a special treat add ½ cup of soy ice cream or sherbet
Blend thoroughly and enjoy!

JOHNNY'S NIRVANIC TEA

Mix equal parts: peppermint
French lavender
licorice root
gotu-kola

Simmer in boiling water for 20 minutes. Strain and serve.

PURPLE SUNSET

1½ cups water
6 mint tea bags, or equivalent in bulk tea
5 cups unsweetened grape juice

2 cups unsweetened apple juice

Steep mint tea in freshly boiled water for 7 minutes, discard bags or remove tea ball and cool.

Mix with juices in 3-quart pitcher, refrigerate if desired.

Mint herb teas mixed with cold apple and other juices become delicious and refreshing drinks.

VEGETABLE BROTH

It is a cleansing and alkalizing drink which supplies a great amount of vitamins and particularly minerals, which are so important for establishing and normalizing a proper chemical balance in the tissues during fasting.

---Paavo Airola, *Are You Confused*

2 large potatoes, unpeeled, chopped into 1/2 –inch pieces
1 cup carrots, shredded or sliced
1 cup beets, shredded or sliced
1 cup celery, leaves included, chopped into ½-inch pieces

Optional: 1 cup any other vegetables—beet tops, turnips & tops, parsley, cabbage, etc.

Put 1½ quarts of water into stainless steel, enamel or earthenware utensil. Slice vegetables directly into the water to prevent oxidations. Cover & cook slowly for ½ hour. Let stand another ½ hour, cool until warm, strain & serve. Keep unused portion in refrigerator and warm to serve.

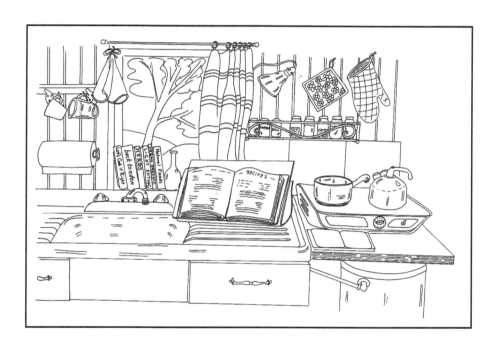

Books & Videos

BOOKS

Airola, Paavo. *Are You Confused?* Phoenix: Health Plus, 1987. Now available via Kindle.

Graham, Sylvester. *A Treatise on Bread, and Bread Making.* Andrews McMeel Publishing, 2012.

Hagler, Louise and Dorothy R. Bates. *The New Farm Vegetarian Cookbook.* Summertown, TN: The Book Publishing Co., 1988.

Harris, Ben Charles. *The Compleat Herbal.* NY: Random House, 1985.

Iyengar, B. K. S. *Light on Yoga.* Rupa HC, 2004.

Kloss, Jethro. *Back to Eden* 2nd edition, Lotus Press, 2004.

Kowalchik, Clair and William Hylton, Eds. Rodale's *Illustrated Encyclopedia of Herbs,* Rodale Books, 1998

Kulvinskas, Viktoras. *Love Your Body.* 21st Century Bookstore, 1972.

------, *Survival into the 21st Century.* Summertown, TN: Book Publishing Company, 2010.

Lappe, Francis Moore. *Diet for a Small Planet.* NY: Ballantine Books, 1992.

Schlosser, Eric. *Fast Food Nation.* Harper Perennial, 2005.

Turner, James. *The Chemical Feast.* NY: Penguin, 1970.

Vishnudevenanda, Swami. *The Complete Illustrated Book of Yoga.* Harmony, 1995.

Vithaldas, Yogi. *The Yoga System of Health and Relief from Tension.* Kessinger Publishing, 2010.

VIDEOS

Food Inc. Director: Robert Kenner. Magnolia Home Entertainment, 2009.

Forks Over Knives. Director: Lee Fulkerson, Virgil Films & Entertainment, 2011.

The Future of Food. Deborah Koons. Garcia Lily Films.

Hungry for Change. Directors: James Colquhoun, Laurentine Ten Bosch, Carlo Ledesma. Docurama, 2012.

Supersize Me. Director: Morgan Spurlock. Sony Pictures, 2004.